M.S. George, H.A. Ring, D.C. Costa,
P.J. Ell, K. Kouris and P.H. Jarritt

# Neuroactivation and Neuroimaging with SPET

Springer-Verlag
London  Berlin  Heidelberg  New York
Paris  Tokyo  Hong Kong
Barcelona  Budapest

Mark S. George, MD
Visiting Research Fellow, Raymond Way Neuropsychiatry Research Group, Department of Clinical Neurology, Institute of Neurology, Queen Square, London, England and Neuropsychiatry Research Fellow, Department of Psychiatry and Behavioral Sciences, Medical University of South Carolina, Charleston, S.C., USA

Howard A. Ring, MRCPsych
Raymond Way Lecturer in Neuropsychiatry, Raymond Way Neuropsychiatry Research Group, Department of Clinical Neurology, Institute of Neurology, Queen Square, London, England

Durval C. Costa, MD, MSc, PhD
Senior Lecturer and Honorary Consultant, Institute of Nuclear Medicine, University College and Middlesex School of Medicine (UCMSM), London, England

Peter J. Ell, MD, MSc, PD, FRCR, FRCP
Professor of Nuclear Medicine, Institute of Nuclear Medicine, University College and Middlesex School of Medicine (UCMSM), London, England

Kypros Kouris, PhD
Lecturer, Institute of Nuclear Medicine, University College and Middlesex School of Medicine (UCMSM), London, England and Associate Professor, University of Kuwait, Kuwait City, Kuwait

Peter H. Jarritt, PhD
Senior Lecturer, Institute of Nuclear Medicine, University College and Middlesex School of Medicine (UCMSM), London, England

ISBN 3-540-19701-X Springer-Verlag Berlin Heidelberg New York
ISBN 0-387-19701-X Springer-Verlag New York Berlin Heidelberg

British Library Cataloguing in Publication Data
Neuroactivation and neuroimaging with SPET
1. Humans. Nervous system. Radiography
I. George, Mark S. *1959–*
616.804757
ISBN 3-540-19701-X

Library of Congress Data available

Apart from any fair dealing for the purposes of research or private study, or criticism or review as permitted under the Copyright, Designs and Patents Act 1988, this publication may only be reproduced, stored or transmitted, in any form or by any means, with the prior permission in writing of the publishers, or in the case of reprographic reproduction in accordance with the terms of licences issued by the Copyright Licensing Agency. Enquiries concerning reproduction outside those terms should be sent to the publishers.

© Springer-Verlag London Limited 1991
Printed in Great Britain

The use of registered names, trademarks etc. in this publication does not imply, even in the absence of a specific statement, that such names are exempt from the relevant laws and regulations and therefore free for general use.

Typeset by Wilmaset, Birkenhead, Wirral
Printed by BAS Printers Limited, Over Wallop, Hampshire
28/3830-543210 Printed on acid-free paper

"Functional changes must not be confounded with pathological changes, although of course the two necessarily co-exist."

*John Hughlings Jackson, 1871*

# Acknowledgements

The authors would like to express their gratitude to the following people and organizations who helped make this book possible:

To the authors' spouses and families for tolerating the long hours away.

To the radiographers at UCMSM for their assistance in obtaining many of the studies used in this book.

To Dr. H. Markus and Dr. C. Katona for supplying information on several of the case examples in Chap. 4.

To Mrs. Gerda McCarthy and the International Autistic Research Foundation for help with the studies on autism.

To Dr. Michael Trimble for his intellectual and emotional support.

To the volunteers who participated in the activation studies and helped advance our working knowledge of SPET imaging and the brain.

To Ciba-Geigy for a travel research grant to Dr. George.

To Mrs. Raymond Way and the Raymond Way Neuropsychiatry Research Fund for financial support to Dr. Ring.

To Amersham International, PLC, for a signficant grant for the application of tracer techniques in neurology and psychiatry.

And to General Electric/CGR for a significant grant towards the development of this project.

# Foreword

Recent explorations in the neurosciences have been progressing towards an understanding of the relationship between brain structure and brain function. Having passed through an era which may be described as one of a localisationist philosophy, in which discrete brain areas were seen to subserve only discrete functions, the perspective of brain–behaviour relationships has advanced in recent years to an appreciation that a more holistic approach is not only heuristically valid, but is also most likely to lead to future advances.

The close relationship between the mind and the brain has been appreciated since the time of Hippocrates when he opined 'men ought to know that from nothing else but thence [from the brain] comes joys, delights, laughter and sports, and sorrows, griefs, despondency and lamentations . . . and by this same organ we become mad and delirious and fears and terrors assail us'. In the nineteenth century, particularly in France and Germany, descriptions of what are now recognised to be independent neurological diseases emerged following empirical clinical observations. Investigation led to the identification in many cases of underlying structural abnormalities which could be linked to pathological changes. Certain neuropsychological symptoms, such as aphasia, were linked with localised brain regions leading to the consolidation of a view of brain–behaviour relationships which was strictly localisationist and relied initially for its confirmation on findings at the post-mortem table. In recent years the advent of neuroimaging as applied to the clinical problems of neurology and psychiatry has led to a re-evaluation of such ideas and to the progressive establishment of new theories. These in turn have been tested with further technological developments.

The era of CT scanning and more recently MRI scanning has allowed such clear anatomical descriptions of the brain to be displayed visually, that some brain–behaviour relationships can be explored in vivo. These will relate entirely to structure. However, the issue of function in relation to structure remains one of the major challenges for the clinical neurosciences. Development of cerebral blood flow analysis used such techniques as inhalation of radioactive nitrous oxide; later xenon was the first stepping stone in what has become a substantial bridge in this field. Although the development of positron emission tomography (PET) is of significant importance, it is still the case that other techniques, and here single photon emission tomography, (also referred to as SPECT) (SPET) comes into its own, have been developing *pari passu* to provide readily accessible alternatives with increasing research and clinical importance.

While it is not the purpose of this text to discuss issues of the relative merits of different technologies, the authors have brought together a succinct document which summarises current work using this state-of-the-art technology. The emphasis here is not on identifying structural change – indeed, to use such investigations for such a purpose would be a redundancy. The point is that alterations of structure which may be shown by some alternative technique can now be inter-linked with functional changes in other regions of the brain. Further, those functional changes can be correlated with behaviour changes. The latter may be an acute paroxysmal state, such as an epileptic ictus or a migraine attack, or a more prolonged behaviour problem, as one might find in a patient with multiple sclerosis, obsessive–compulsive disorder or schizophrenia.

The brain as envisaged by neuroscientists as we approach the turn of the century is not that of the brain carefully dissected by the nineteenth-century pathologists, nor even that of the neuroanatomy lessons of those of us who went to medical school in the 1950s and 60s. Theories of neuronal function have progressed rapidly, taking into account a multitude of factors which have emerged from new neuroanatomical techniques that have allowed neurochemical pathways to be identified which interlink hitherto apparently discrete and separate brain regions with one another. These, in vivo, are best identified by functional imaging.

An exciting era is just emerging with the concept of activation techniques, the idea being to examine, in both healthy and diseased brains, how the latter respond to environmental challenges. These may be as simple as the repetitive movement of the fingers of one hand to more complex cognitive problem solving. These techniques are explored in this book and the possibilities that they will bring for future understanding of the consequences of cerebral disease in neurology and psychiatry become obvious. Interpretation of the results of these findings must be seen alongside developing concepts of how the brain works, the latter constantly changing in the light of the results of investigations such as are being carried out by the group that have produced this book.

For those less interested in the more esoteric aspects of either brain scanning or parallel distributed processing the atlas itself provides a glorious Technicolor view of the living human brain in health and disease. We can only wonder what Hughlings Jackson or Gowers would have made of the exciting progress which has been made in the neurosciences in recent years.

London,  
1991

Michael R. Trimble  
FRCP, FRCPsych

# Contents

**Foreword** by Michael R. Trimble, FRCP, FRCPsych . . . . . ix

**Part I: Functional Neuroimaging with Radioactive Tracers** . . . . . . . . . . . . . . . . . . . . . . . . . . . 1

  1 Principles of Emission Tomography . . . . . . . . . . . 3
  2 Radiopharmaceutical Ligands and Tracers . . . . . . . . . 11
  3 SPET Instrumentation: Characteristics and New Developments . . . . . . . . . . . . . . . . . . . . . 29
  4 Clinical Use of SPET Imaging in Psychiatric and Neurological Disease . . . . . . . . . . . . . . . . . . 51

**Part II: Neuroactivation with SPET** . . . . . . . . . . . 121

  5 A Historical and Philosophical Review of Localizing Brain Function . . . . . . . . . . . . . . . . . . . . . . . 123
  6 Models of Brain Processing with Respect to Functional Neuroimaging . . . . . . . . . . . . . . . . . . . . . 133
  7 Description and Principles of Neuroactivation . . . . . . 143
  8 Review of Previous SPET Neuroactivation Studies in Normal Controls . . . . . . . . . . . . . . . . . . . . 153
  9 Activation Protocols in Normal Subjects Using SPET: A Window into Normal Brain Function . . . . . . . . . . 157
 10 Activation Studies in Specific Disease States: Future Applications . . . . . . . . . . . . . . . . . . . . . 173

**Appendixes:**
  I Area-Specific Activation Tasks . . . . . . . . . . . . . 183
 II A Guide to Performing Neuroactivation Studies . . . . . 184

**Selected Bibliography** . . . . . . . . . . . . . . . . . . 185

**Subject Index** . . . . . . . . . . . . . . . . . . . . . . 193

*Part I:*

# Functional Neuroimaging with Radioactive Tracers

Chapter 1
# Principles of Emission Tomography

## Introduction

Medical radionuclide imaging involves the administration to a patient of an appropriate radionuclide linked to a specific pharmaceutical. Most radionuclides used for medical imaging purposes fall into two broad categories (Tables 1 and 2): (a) Single photon emitters: radionuclides that predominantly emit gamma or X-rays with energies usually varying between 80 and 360 keV; (b) positron emitters: radionuclides that emit positrons which essentially behave like positive electrons. After colliding with neighbouring electrons, thereby losing its kinetic energy, the positron (now at rest or almost at rest) unites with an electron in a process called positron-electron annihilation, which results in the emission of two gamma rays of 511 keV energy, travelling in almost opposite directions. Whether with single photon or with positron emitters, the imaging process relies on the detection of emitted gamma rays. A position-

**Table 1.** Radionuclides for SPET

|         | keV      | Half-life (hours) |
|---------|----------|-------------------|
| $^{99m}$Tc | 140      | 6.0               |
| $^{123}$I  | 159      | 13.2              |
| $^{111}$In | 171, 245 | 67.3              |
| $^{201}$Tl | 68–82    | 73.1              |
| $^{133}$Xe | 81       | 126.0             |

**Table 2.** Radionuclides for PET

|         | keV | Half-life (min) |
|---------|-----|-----------------|
| $^{82}$Rb  | 511 | 1.25            |
| $^{15}$O   | 511 | 2.0             |
| $^{13}$N   | 511 | 10.0            |
| $^{11}$C   | 511 | 20.0            |
| $^{68}$Ga  | 511 | 68.0            |
| $^{18}$F   | 511 | 111.0           |

and energy-sensitive radiation detector is used, coupled to a computer system which controls the data acquisition and performs the data processing.

Starting from the general principle of imaging, this chapter provides an introduction to tomographic imaging with both single-photon emitters (single-photon emission tomography: SPET) and positron emitters (positron emission tomography: PET). Emphasis is on SPET. Both SPET and PET are placed within the context of other tomographic imaging modalities.

## Planar Emission Imaging

Single photon emitting radionuclides have been used to label radiopharmaceuticals since the late 1950s. The most important development came with the discovery of technetium-99m ($^{99m}$Tc) by Harper et al. (1962). $^{99m}$Tc is now used in almost 90% of all diagnostic imaging procedures carried out in nuclear medicine. The almost universally used radiation detector for these studies is the Anger gamma camera introduced by Anger (1958). It basically consists of a collimator, a sodium iodide NaI(Tl) scintillation crystal, an array of photomultiplier tubes (PMTs), and associated electronics. The gamma rays emitted from the patient are detected by the gamma camera, leading to image formation.

With visible light, an image is formed using mirrors and lenses that bend and focus the light photons, thereby guiding them along a precise path on to a recording device. Gamma rays cannot be focused in the optical sense, but for an image to be formed a similar principle must be obeyed, namely that there must be a one-to-one correspondence between the direction of emission of a gamma ray and its point of detection (Kouris et al. 1982). The collimator in single-photon imaging and the electronic collimation of the annihilation gamma rays in positron imaging are the means for achieving this requirement.

In gamma-camera imaging, the collimator is a large plate of lead with literally thousands of small holes placed in front of the crystal between the patient and the crystal. Only gamma rays travelling through the collimator holes may contribute to image formation. Unfortunately, most of the gamma rays emitted during the data acquisition time do not travel in the direction(s) allowed by the collimator(s) and therefore do not contribute to image formation. It is in this sense that radionuclide imaging is a photon-limited process. For single-photon imaging, typically only 1 in about $10^5$ emitted gamma rays is detected. The scintillation crystal transforms the imaging gamma rays into light photons. These are collected by the photomultiplier tubes, which then generate a measurable current. The associated electronic circuitry processes the pulses from the PMTs, computes the energy and location ('point') of detection of each gamma ray and feeds the information to a computer for image display, processing and storage.

In planar radionuclide imaging using a gamma camera, the three-dimensional (3D) distribution of activity in the organ or tissue of interest is represented as a two-dimensional (2D) image called a view or projection in a specified direction. Each point on the image has a value equal to (or an intensity level proportional to) the sum of the gamma rays detected by the NaI(Tl) crystal at the corresponding point. For these gamma rays to have been detected, they must have travelled through the corresponding collimator hole which, in the case of a parallel hole collimator, is perpendicular to the face of the gamma camera. The view or projection referred to above is then said to be obtained along this direction. In the absence of scattering in the tissue, the detection of a gamma ray would convey the information that a radiopharmaceutical molecule had existed somewhere along the line going through the collimator hole and that it disintegrated during the measurement time interval. The position, i.e. the depth, of the labelled molecule along the line is not known, and it is in this sense that the measurement of all the gamma rays in this direction is a projection.

## Emission Tomography

The aim of any tomographic imaging method is to obtain information, formatted into an image from a well-defined section of tomogram of the patient (brain or body). Once this is achieved, the information contained in such a tomogram is inherently in three dimensions – a tomogram has a defined thickness, length and width. This is in contrast to conventional planar imaging where the information from any depth is superimposed onto two dimensions. With a series of images of sequential slices, full 3D visualization of the organ or tissue of interest can be achieved.

Essentially, in order to obtain an image of a slice with any tomographic method, data must be acquired in a multitude of directions and then processed by a computer that performs image reconstruction (Herman 1980). The data are measurements that reflect how the physical parameter of interest (e.g. density reflecting anatomy or activity concentration reflecting physiology) varies along each one of these lines. Conceptually, this may be understood as building up information about the internal structure or distribution of interest by viewing the region externally through an information carrier that can traverse the body or part of the body along different directions.

In order to obtain a tomogram with SPET, the organ to be studied is 'viewed' by a detector and data are acquired over a wide range of angles. In the early 1970s, the Anger gamma camera was mounted onto a circular gantry, allowing the detector to rotate around the organ or patient to be scanned. Thus, SPET became available as a new diagnostic imaging methodology (Williams 1985). A description of other attempts at SPET with different types of instrumentation falls outside the scope of this monograph, but the interested reader will find useful references at the the end of this chapter (Ell and Holman 1982; Williams 1985).

The most common device for SPET is the single rotating Anger-type gamma camera fitted with a parallel-hole collimator. When it rotates through 360°, full-angle tomography is obtained. This is a prerequisite for most SPET studies when the best tomographic detail and sharpness (resolution) and signal differentiation (contrast) is to be obtained. In specific circumstances, the camera rotates through 180° only. A typical example is seen in tomographic imaging of the distribution of myocardial perfusion with thallium-201 ($^{201}$Tl) chloride. In other circumstances, using different instrumentation, a narrower range of angles is scanned, and this is referred to as limited or narrow-angle tomography. The reasons for such choices will not be discussed here – suffice it to state that for the brain, almost all imaging procedures view this organ from a complete 360° rotation.

With the patient remaining still, the gamma camera records data usually at approximately 3–6° increments. For each of these increments, a planar image called a view or projection is obtained and stored by the computer. How this process is then converted into a tomogram, is explained in Chap. 3. Systems with more than one camera on a rotating gantry or with an array of detectors have been introduced in order to increase the number of lines along which gamma rays can be detected, thereby increasing the efficiency of the imaging process. The reconstructed resolution can also improve if high-resolution collimators are used. A detailed description of these systems is given in Chap. 3.

In PET, the fundamental measurement defining a 'line' is a coincidence event, i.e. the simultaneous detection of the two gamma rays emitted as a result of a positron-electron annihilation. For each line, two opposing detectors are required to be connected in electronic coincidence. The most common device for PET comprises an array of detectors forming a ring and collecting coincidence events from one slice. Adjacent rings collect data from adjacent and interleaving slices with or without the use of collimators for slice definition. Further discussion of PET instrumentation and applications is outside the scope of this book, but the interested reader will find relevant references at the end of this chapter (Kouris et al. 1982; Phelps et al. 1986).

As stated earlier, the objective of tomography is to provide 3D visualization of the organ or tissue of interest. Single-slice machines provide an image of only one tomographic slice at a time. More commonly with multislice machines, data are acquired which enable the reconstruction of a series of thin consecutive slices spanning the entire region. The reconstructed image of each slice is a matrix ($N \times N$) of pixels. With M slices present, the reconstructed pixels form a 3D array of numbers ($N \times N \times M$), which can be mathematically manipulated to give slices in any desired direction. With the patient usually supine, the original reconstructed slices are commonly transaxial. If M is sufficiently large, one can directly obtain the coronal and sagittal slices. Oblique slices in other desirable directions would require data interpolation.

Image quality is governed by how well the imaging system physically achieves the above principle of correspondence between the direction of gamma ray emission and the point of detection. This is dependent on the design of the collimator, which in turn defines the 'lines', and on the precision with which the detector locates the 'point' of detection. Another factor governing image quality is gamma-ray scattering within the tissue since each scattered gamma ray will provide the wrong spatial information if it is detected with sufficient energy. The total number of gamma rays detected is also crucial to image quality since radioactive decay is a random process governed by Poisson statistics. The greater the number of gamma rays used the better because statistical fluctuations will be reduced, but patient comfort and movement impose practical restrictions.

A large number of radiopharmaceuticals have been developed for use in man labelled with single-photon or positron-emitting radionuclides, (Tables 3 and 4). Each radiopharmaceutical is designed to permit the investigation of specific organ functions. A detailed description of the radiopharmaceuticals developed for SPET and PET is not intended here. The reader is referred to specific references in this expanding field (Ell 1990; Kilbourn 1990; Verbruggen 1990). However, a more detailed description of radiopharmaceuticals relevant to brain SPET is the subject of Chap. 2 of this book.

Table 3. Typical radiopharmaceuticals for SPET

| Radiopharmaceutical | To study |
| --- | --- |
| $^{99m}$Tc-HMPAO | Cerebral blood flow |
| $^{99m}$Tc-MDP | Skeletal metabolism |
| $^{201}$Tl-chloride | Myocardial perfusion |
| $^{123}$I-IBZM | Dopamine D-2 receptor |

HMPAO, Hexamethylpropylene amine oxime; MDP, methylene diphosphonate; IBZM, iodobenzamide

Table 4. Typical radiopharmaceuticals for PET

| Radiopharmaceutical | To study |
| --- | --- |
| $^{18}$F-deoxyglucose | Cerebral metabolism |
| $^{11}$C-methionine | Amino acid turnover |
| $^{15}$O-oxygen | Metabolism |
| $^{11}$C-dopamine | Dopamine receptor system |

# Other Tomographic Imaging Modalities

With SPET and PET, tomographic imaging reflects the interactions of the administered radiopharmaceutical and the organ or tissue under investigation, and hence in vivo autoradiography is achieved.

True 3D tomographic imaging is also achieved by computed X-ray transmission tomography (CT scanning) and by nuclear magnetic resonance imaging (MRI scanning). While for SPET and PET radiation emitted from the patient is used (emission tomography), for CT X-rays are generated externally and then transmitted through the body (transmission tomography). MRI is a process of resonant absorption and re-emission of radiofrequency energy in the presence of externally applied magnetic fields.

SPET and PET have been developed to offer different information to CT and MRI. While SPET and PET primarily depict functional and/or metabolic information, X-ray CT and MRI offer exquisite anatomical and morphological detail. Hence, it is clear that these different imaging modalities are complementary. A comparison of their capabilities in terms of spatial resolution and minimum detectable quantities is given in Tables 5 and 6.

Tables 5 and 6 clearly demonstrate why CT and MRI excel in the demonstration of anatomical detail (in view of their superior spatial resolution).

**Table 5.** Spatial resolution (mm)

| CT  | MRI | PET | SPET |
|-----|-----|-----|------|
| 1–2 | 1–2 | 3–5 | 6–10 |

**Table 6.** Minimum detectable quantities

| $10^{-3}$ g | orders of magnitude | | $10^{-12}$ g |
|---|---|---|---|
| mg | µg | ng | pg |
| CT/MRI ← | | | → SPET/PET |

However, SPET and PET excel in the recording of functional and/or metabolic information through the specific imaging of a range of biologically relevant radiopharmaceuticals and the application of tracer methodology. It is the high signal derived from minute quantities of the administered radionuclide which permits SPET and PET to carry out studies of the blood-brain barrier, brain blood flow, dopamine receptor system and other neuroreceptor systems.

# Radiation Exposure

While MRI imaging does not involve any ionizing radiation, X-ray CT, SPET and PET do expose the patient to a certain amount of radiation. The amount of radiation to which the patient is exposed should be the lowest required to provide an adequate quality study in accordance with the radiation protection principle ALARA (as low as reasonable achievable) (ICRP 1988). Table 7 gives typical radiation exposure values expressed as effective dose equivalent (EDE) for the study of the brain (ICRP 1988; DoH 1988). Table 8 gives data for other imaging procedures for comparative purposes.

**Table 7.** Typical radiation exposure (I)

|  | EDE (mSv) |
|---|---|
| X-ray CT brain scan (without contrast) | 3 |
| SPET blood-brain-barrier scan (800 MBq pertechnetate) | 10 |
| SPET cerebral blood flow scan (555 MBq $^{99m}$Tc-HMPAO) | 7.6 |
| SPET $^{123}$I-IBZM (185 MBq) | 3.6 |
| PET $^{18}$FDG scan (370 MBq) | 10 |

HMPAO, Hexamethylpropylene amine oxime; IBZM, iodobenzamide; FDG, fluorodeoxyglucose; EDE, effective dose equivalent

Table 8. Typical radiation exposure (II)

|  | EDE (mSv) |
|---|---|
| Chest X-ray | 0.05–0.1 |
| Abdomen CT | 3–9 |
| Barium enema | 7.7 |
| IVP | 4.4 |

# References

Anger HO (1958) Scintillation camera. Rev Sci Instrum 29:27–33
DoH Publication (1988) Notes for guidance on the administration of radioactive substances to persons for the purposes of diagnosis, treatment or research. DoH, London
Ell PJ (1990) Highlights of the European Association of Nuclear Medicine Congress, Amsterdam 1990. Eur J Nucl Med 17:873–891
Ell PJ, Holman BL (eds) (1982) Computed emission tomography. Oxford Medical Publications, Oxford
Harper PV, Andros G, Lathrop K (1962) Preliminary observations on the use of six-hour $Tc^{99m}$ as a tracer in biology and medicine. Argonne Cancer Research Hospital Semiannual Report to the Atomic Energy Commission, no. 18. Office of Technical Services, Department of Commerce, Washington, DC, pp 76–88
Herman GT (1980) Image reconstruction from projections: the fundamentals of computerized tomography. Academic Press, London
ICRP Publication 53 (1988) Radiation dose to patients from radiopharmaceuticals. Annals of the ICRP, Pergamon Press, Oxford
Kilbourn MR (1990) Fluorine-18 labeling of radiopharmaceuticals. Nuclear Medicine Science series, NAS-NS-3203. National Academy Press, Washington, DC
Kouris K, Spyrou NM, Jackson DF (1982) Imaging with ionizing radiations. Surrey University Press, Blackie & Son, Glasgow
Phelps ME, Maziota JC, Schelbert HR (1986) Positron emission tomography and autoradiography. Raven Press, New York
Verbruggen A (1990) Radiopharmaceuticals: state of the art. Eur J Nucl Med 17:346–364
Williams ED (ed) (1985) An introduction to emission computed tomography. Report no. 44. Institute of Physical Sciences in Medicine, London

Chapter 2
# Radiopharmaceutical Ligands and Tracers

## Introduction

In recent years improvements in instrumentation and radiopharmaceutical developments have broadened the scope of single-photon emission tomography (SPET) of the brain. Patients with neurological and psychiatric diseases may be better assessed. More objective parameters (i.e. brain perfusion, neuroreceptor availability, neurotransmitter utilization) can now be used to study the natural progression of disease and to determine its response to either established or new therapeutic interventions.

This progress has almost obscured the merits of past conventional blood-brain barrier (BBB) imaging with radiotracers. These have been in use for more than three decades to diagnose disruption in the BBB but have become a second port of call with the advent of computer-assisted X-ray tomography (CT) and magnetic resonance imaging (MRI). Conventional BBB tracers still play an important role in patient management, particularly because of the ease of use, wide availability and low cost.

The BBB appears to be a limiting step for the uptake of all radiotracers in the brain. The aim of this chapter is to describe briefly the structural components underlying the BBB and to give an account of the different possibilities of imaging normal and diseased brain with radiopharmaceuticals.

## The Blood-Brain Barrier

The BBB is a functional concept that identifies the special permeability characteristics of a microstructure composed of endothelial and glial cells. All capillaries within the central nervous system are lined with endothelial cells without gaps between them. The blood in the capillary lumen is separated from the neurons by the endothelial cells with their basement membrane and surrounded by multiple astrocytic processes (Fig. 1). The arrangement of this complex structure is such that there is little space for the small amount of extracellular water (20% of total brain water, corresponding to 25% of total brain weight). This structure, consisting of endothelial cells, basement membrane and perivascular astrocytic processes, is named the BBB. Its main

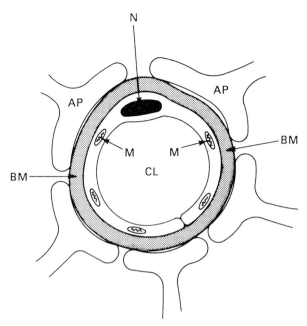

**Fig 1.** Structural components of the blood-brain barrier. *AP*, Astrocytic process; *BM*, basement membrane; *CL*, capillary lumen; *M*, mitochondria; *N*, Nucleus.

function is to regulate the passage of solutes, nutrients and other chemicals transported in the plasma.

When a dye (such as trypan blue) is administered intravenously to a mammal, staining of the perivascular astrocytic processes is seen. The neurons are spared, except for areas of the brain where the BBB is either incomplete (pineal, pituitary, area postrema of the brain stem, choroid plexus and locus coeruleus: Dempsey and Wislocki 1955) or disrupted.

Although the intact BBB is not permeable to large molecules (Reese and Karnovsky 1968), gases, water, glucose, electrolytes and amino acids can pass across this barrier into the neurons and extracellular space. Different mechanisms (Bradbury 1985) preside over this passage through the BBB: (1) passive diffusion (water, gases); (2) facilitated transport (amino-acids); (3) active transport (glucose).

Trauma, inflammatory processes and/or cerebrovascular insults may cause rupture of the BBB with consequent disorganization of its permeability properties. Therefore, intra- and extracellular concentrations of water, electrolytes and proteins may change significantly (Miller and Hess 1958).

Two main groups of radiotracers are used for neuroimaging. The first group consists of those tracers that are not capable of crossing the normal BBB. They are often referred to as the conventional BBB radiotracers: technetium-99m ($^{99m}$Tc) pertechnetate, $^{99m}$Tc-diethylene triamine penta-acetic acid (DTPA), $^{99m}$Tc-glucoheptonate (GH) and $^{201}$Tl as thallous chloride. The other group is composed of radiotracers with different degrees of lipophilicity. They either diffuse passively or are easily transported across the BBB. The latter are mainly subdivided into two other groups: perfusion tracers ($^{123}$I-iodoamphetamine

(IMP), $^{123}$I-hydroxymethyliodobenzyldiamine (HIPDM), $^{99m}$Tc-hexamethylpropylene amine oxime (HMPAO), $^{99m}$Tc-ethyl cysteinate dimer (ECD), $^{99m}$Tc-boric acid adducts of technetium oximes (BATO-2 MP)) and neuroreceptor ligands ($^{123}$I-flumazenil, $^{123}$I-iodobenzamide (IBZM), $^{123}$I-ketanserin, $^{123}$I-(R)-3-quinuclidinyl-4-iodo-benzilate (IQNB)).

## Radiopharmaceuticals: Blood-Brain Barrier

In the early 1970s, $^{99m}$Tc-pertechnetate was widely used. Mainly planar imaging of the brain (Maynard et al. 1969; DeLand 1971) was undertaken in order to detect intracranial lesions causing breakdown of the BBB. Cerebrovascular disease (Glasco et al. 1965; Fischer and Miale 1972), intracerebral tumours (White et al. 1976) and intracranial haematomas (Hopkins and Kristensen 1973) were identified and their intracranial localization assessed with multiple projections.

The advent of X-ray computed tomography (CT scan: Hounsfield 1973; Baker et al. 1974) also led to a refinement of the radionuclide brain-imaging technique. New radiopharmaceuticals (Waxman et al. 1976; Rollo et al. 1977; Ryerson et al. 1978) and tomography (Carril et al. 1979; Ell et al. 1980; Hill et al. 1980) were put to use. These significantly improved the sensitivity (Carril et al. 1979) and specificity of detection of cerebrovascular disease and intracerebral tumours (Ell et al. 1980; Hill et al. 1980).

$^{99m}$Tc-pertechnetate has a number of important advantages. These include availability, almost ideal physical properties for imaging, a short effective half-life and favourable radiation dosimetry. With experience some disadvantages were identified. These included a relatively slow clearance from blood and uptake by other organs such as the salivary glands and the choroid plexus.

$^{99m}$Tc-labelled DTPA and $^{99m}$Tc-GH are more rapidly excreted (DTPA by the kidneys and GH by the kidneys and hepatobiliary system), hence significantly reducing the signal from background blood-pool. Lesions were seen with higher contrast resolution, further improved by using SPET. Table 1 shows $^{99m}$Tc-GH as the BBB radiotracer of choice. Its cost is similar to others, the tracer radiation dosimetry is more favourable than that of $^{99m}$Tc-pertechnetate and its blood clearance is faster than the other two. Interestingly, it was shown that uptake in tumours mimicked that of glucose (Rollo et al. 1977).

The use of these BBB radiotracers is nowadays restricted to the detection of

Table 1. Relative merits of conventional blood-brain barrier radiotracers

|  | Pertechnetate | DTPA | GH |
| --- | --- | --- | --- |
| Cost[a] | 1 | 1 | 1 |
| Blood clearance | Slow | Fast | Faster |
| Imaging time (post-injection) | 1–3 h | 2–3 h | 1–1.5 h |
| EDE[b] (mSv/MBq) | 0.013 | 0.0063 | 0.009 |
| (mSv/500 MBq) | 6.5 | 3.2 | 4.5 |

[a]From Clarke et al. (1990); large variations are likely
[b]EDE, Effective dose equivalent (manufacturer's information)

intracerebral secondary deposits where CT and MRI are not immediately available. Their accuracy for distinguishing tumour recurrence from post-radiation necrosis is poor, because all (conventional BBB tracers, iodinated contrast for CT scan and gadolinium for MRI) rely on a breakdown of the BBB.

Recently, $^{201}$Tl-thallous chloride has been reported to be a useful radiopharmaceutical for the pre-operative evaluation of patients with brain tumours (Kim et al. 1990). In a series of 29 patients $^{201}$Tl-thallous chloride was superior to CT scan, $^{99m}$Tc-GH and $^{67}$Ga-citrate for identifying variable recurrent tumours. In this work and other reports (Mountz et al. 1988; Black et al 1989; Kaplan et al. 1989), relative quantification of tumour $^{201}$Tl uptake demonstrated statistically significant differences between low-grade and high-grade tumours. This is explained by the uptake mechanism in tumour cells, which is based upon the sodium-potassium pump (ATPase) in the cell membrane. In addition, its uptake is higher in cells with faster growth rates. In the brain $^{201}$Tl is taken up by active tumour cells and not by normal cells, oedematous tissue or necrotic areas (Gruber and Hochberg 1990).

Further prospective studies are still required to evaluate the accuracy and sensitivity of $^{201}$Tl SPET of the brain for the pre-, post-operative and in particular, post-irradiation therapy assessment of patients with brain tumours.

A completely different mechanism has been described for the uptake of L-3-$^{123}$I-iodomethyltyrosine ($^{123}$I-IMT), another brain tumour marker (Biersack et al. 1989). It uses the amino-acid-facilitated transport system to cross the BBB and shows a tumour uptake comparable with that of $^{11}$C-labelled amino acids, without being incorporated into proteins. It is a potentially useful radioactive tracer for imaging brain tumours and studying amino acid utilization by tumour cells.

## Radiopharmaceuticals: Cerebral Blood Volume

It is possible to label red bloods cells (r.b.c.) with stannous chloride and $^{99m}$Tc using either an in vivo or an in vitro method. Labelled r.b.c. given intravenously permits the study of total or regional blood volume. With this radiopharmaceutical it is possible to detect sites of bleeding and to study regional blood volume in the meninges, brain and brain tumours. It has been used specifically to assess brain perfusion reserve when associated with the study of regional cerebral blood flow (Knapp et al. 1986).

The plasma volume of the brain may be calculated if either $^{123}$I- or $^{99m}$Tc-labelled human serum albumin (HSA) is used and SPET undertaken. A reasonable estimate of the regional brain haematocrit may then be calculated by combining r.b.c. and HSA studies.

## Radiopharmaceuticals: Brain Perfusion

In general, lipophilic compounds with a neutral charge pass through the intact BBB and reach the neurons of the cortical and subcortical structures of the

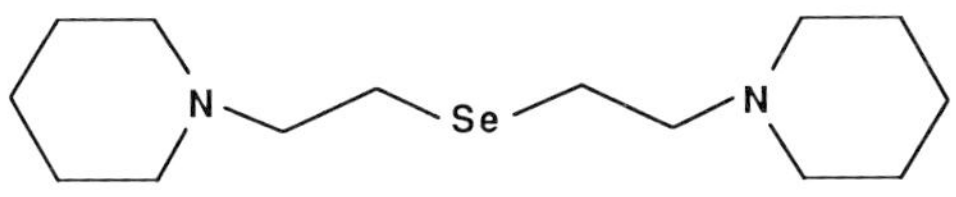

**PIPSE**

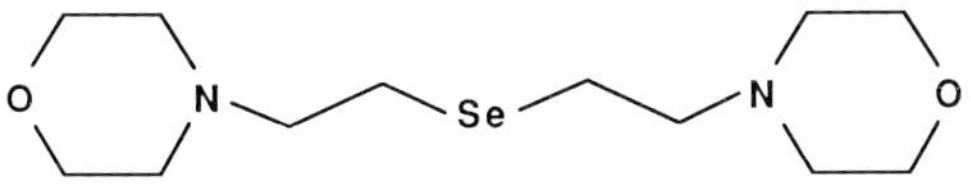

**MOSE**

**Fig 2.** Chemical structures of PIPSE and MOSE.

brain. In order to be used for brain perfusion studies, these tracers have to meet several criteria: they must be able to pass through the intact BBB, they must have a high (first-pass) extraction efficiency with no significant redistribution, they must exhibit prolonged retention in the brain to allow for SPET, they must have an effective regional distribution in the brain proportional to the regional distribution of blood flow rates to the different cortical and subcortical structures, and finally they must have little or no metabolism.

After the initial description of selenium-75-labelled diamines (Kung and Blau 1980), MOSE and PIPSE (Fig. 2), all effort has been directed towards the development of $^{123}$I, and particularly $^{99m}$Tc-labelled brain perfusion radiotracers.

## $^{123}$I-Labelled Amines

The first iodinated amine reported in the literature that was capable of measuring regional brain perfusion was $^{123}$I-iodoantipyrine (Uzler et al. 1975). It is lipophilic and therefore crosses the intact BBB. Since it diffuses passively through the cell membrane and exhibits no retention mechanism, $^{123}$I-iodoantipyrine washes out from the brain quickly. SPET is hence impracticable. Two other amine derivatives emerged later. One is a monoamine, N-isopropyl[$^{123}$I]-p-iodo-amphetamine ($^{123}$I-IMP) and the other a diamine, $^{123}$I-HIPDM:[$^{123}$I]N,N,N'-trimethyl-n '-[2-hydroxy-3-methyl-5-iodobenzyl]-1,3-propane diamine. Figure 3 shows the chemical structure of these tracers. $^{123}$I-IMP was approved by the Food and Drug Administration in 1988.

The mechanism of uptake and retention in the brain is very similar for both tracers and is thought to be a function of: metabolism of the primary amine into a non-lipophilic form, possibly by demethylation via N-methyl transferase; retention in intracellular organelles, such as the lysosomes, receptor or protein binding.

It was initially proposed that a pH shift gradient mechanism is present so that, once inside the cell, the primary compound is submitted to a sudden

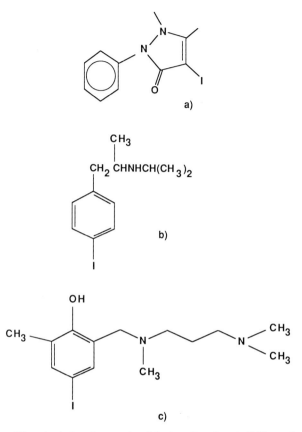

**Fig 3a–c.** Chemical structures of **a** 4-iodoantipyrine, **b** IMP, and **c** HIPDM.

change in pH that converts the amine into a non-lipophilic cation. However, this assumption is questionable.

The kinetics of these tracers are very similar, as is their biodistribution in man. Both tracers are initially accumulated in the lungs and have similar lung-clearance profiles. Brain uptake is 30-40% higher for $^{123}$I-IMP than $^{123}$I-HIPDM. The rate of brain uptake is faster for $^{123}$I-HIPDM. At 2 min post-injection 75% of the maximum brain uptake is achieved with $^{123}$I-HIPDM compared to only 45% with $^{123}$I-IMP. Later on, between 30 min and 1 h post-injection, the brain radioactivity for both is unchanged and enables SPET to be carried out. The regional distribution of the two radiotracers is similar between 20 and 60 min post-injection. Liver uptake is higher for the monoamine than for the diamine. $^{123}$I-HIPDM concentrates in the pancreas with a 11:1 percent injected dose per gram ratio between the pancreas and the liver.

After 60 min post-injection these amines are redistributed into the brain. The initial distribution in the brain, which is proportional to the regional distribution of perfusion and cerebral blood flow, is lost. In cases of acute 'stroke', the initial image shows a photon deficiency in the area of vascular insult that is 'filled in' by amine metabolites from the lungs. It is said that this late

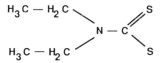

Fig 4. Chemical structure of DDC (diethyldithiocarbamate).

redistribution may be representative of cerebral tissue viability linked to the presence of catecholamine receptors.

While considerable experience has been obtained with these radiopharmaceuticals, labelling with $^{123}$I precludes their use on a daily basis.

## $^{201}$Tl- Diethyldithiocarbamate

Sodium diethyldithiocarbamate (NaDDC) is a metabolite of disulfiram that binds easily to metallic ions. It has been clinically used to treat nickel poisoning, thallium intoxication and Wilson's disease. During the treatment of thallium intoxication patients sometimes develop more neurological symptoms that are worse than those from the intoxication. This is explained by the increased lipophilic status of the resulting chelate, $^{201}$Tl-DDC (Fig. 4). This incidental finding led to pharmacokinetic experiments in rats that demonstrated that an approximately ten-fold increase in brain uptake is obtained with $^{201}$Tl-DDC in comparison to $^{201}$Tl-thallous chloride (Vyth et al. 1983).

Studies in man (Van Royen et al. 1987) have demonstrated a first-pass brain extraction reaching a plateau by 90 s post-injection with no further redistribution. Its distribution in the human body follows the relative distribution of the cardiac output. The tracer has rapid clearance from the lungs. By 5 min, the radioactivity in the lungs falls to 45% of the initial lung peak value. $^{201}$Tl-DDC is excreted through the kidneys and the hepatobiliary system.

$^{201}$Tl-DDC can be used to study acute disease (ictus, stroke). With its long physical half-life (78 h) patients can be scanned several hours after the acute event. The CBF/SPET study still reflects CBF at the time of administration. Image quality is, however, suboptimal. There is significant attenuation of the low energy (78 keV) photons.

## $^{99m}$Tc-Labelled Tracers

For nuclear medicine studies to be carried out in a routine environment, tracers have to be available 5 days a week without supply or distribution difficulties. For this reason, tracers labelled with $^{99m}$Tc represent up to 85% of all nuclear medicine procedures carried out worldwide.

$^{99m}$Tc is supplied from a generator system that is delivered weekly to thousands of hospitals. When eluting this generator with saline, large quantities of $^{99m}$Tc-pertechnetate are obtained in a sterile, pyrogen-free vial.

The knowledge that metabolism 'drives' flow and remains coupled with it in the greater majority of circumstances (the typical known exception is the entity of acute stroke in the first few hours of the event) adds weight to the pursuit of a tracer that depicts the distribution of flow/perfusion in the brain, while being labelled with the ubiquitous $^{99m}$Tc radionuclide.

It is worth remembering that such tracers will permit the investigation of disease with a high prevalence and significant social and economic consequences. As an example, cerebrovascular disease is the third-most-common cause of death in the USA and Europe. The annual incidence of stroke rises with age and is greater than 1% per year in those over 65 years old. The natural history of the disease is not well understood and medical management is often subjective and too dependent on clinical criteria alone. A second example can be given in the context of the study of dementia. Between 3% and 5% of individuals over the age of 65 suffer from impairment of memory, personality changes and mild dementia. Senile dementia is present in less than 1% of people under the age of 65, and it rises to more than 15% in those over 85. There is a clear age dependency for dementia, and the prevalence of this condition is growing as the percentage of elderly persons in the population at large increases.

Returning to the general requirements for a clinically useful tracer for CBF and SPET studies, the $^{99m}$Tc-labelled tracer should: be electrically neutral and lipophilic to enable passive diffusion across the intact BBB; exhibit a high extraction efficiency (in order to be distributed in the brain primarily mediated by flow during its first passage through the cerebral circulation); remain trapped inside the brain for sufficient time to allow its detection by the imaging process.

Other considerations are also taken into account when choosing such a tracer: chemical stability, ease of preparation, dosimetry and cost. Cost is often determined by the number of individual patient doses that can be extracted from any single vial. This if often achievable despite the restrictive advice some manufacturers give.

In the development of these tracers a breakthrough occurred with the synthesis at Amersham Laboratories, UK, of a series of amine derivatives of propylene amine oxime (PnAO). The first clinical studies with $^{99m}$Tc-HMPAO were carried out at the Institute of Nuclear Medicine, UCMSM, in 1985 (Ell et al. 1985). These confirmed that HMPAO offered almost optimal characteristics for clinical cerebral blood flow (CBF) SPET studies in man (Costa et al. 1986). All CBF SPET studies presented in this book were carried out with this tracer.

Since the discovery of $^{99m}$Tc-HMPAO, a number of other tracers have become available and have been submitted to extensive experimental, animal and also human testing. The structures of the most relevant CBF tracers labelled with $^{99m}$Tc are shown in Fig. 5, and Tables 2 and 3 show comparative data for these compounds that have reached the stage of commercial exploitation (Verbruggen 1990).

$^{99m}$Tc-L,L-ECD (DuPont) exhibits rapid blood clearance and urinary excretion. The compound is rapidly converted by the liver to a polar bi-acid metabolite (Leveille et al. 1989; Siccardi et al. 1989). Due to this rapid excretion, the radiation exposure from this compound is significantly reduced (Van Nerom et al. 1990).

$^{99m}$Tc-MRP 20 (Medgenix) belongs to a new class of tetradentate-complexing agents, characterized by the presence of a pyrrole and azomethine moiety in their structure (Libson et al. 1989). As stated by Verbruggen in his seminal review on $^{99m}$Tc-radiopharmaceuticals (Verbruggen 1990) these compounds

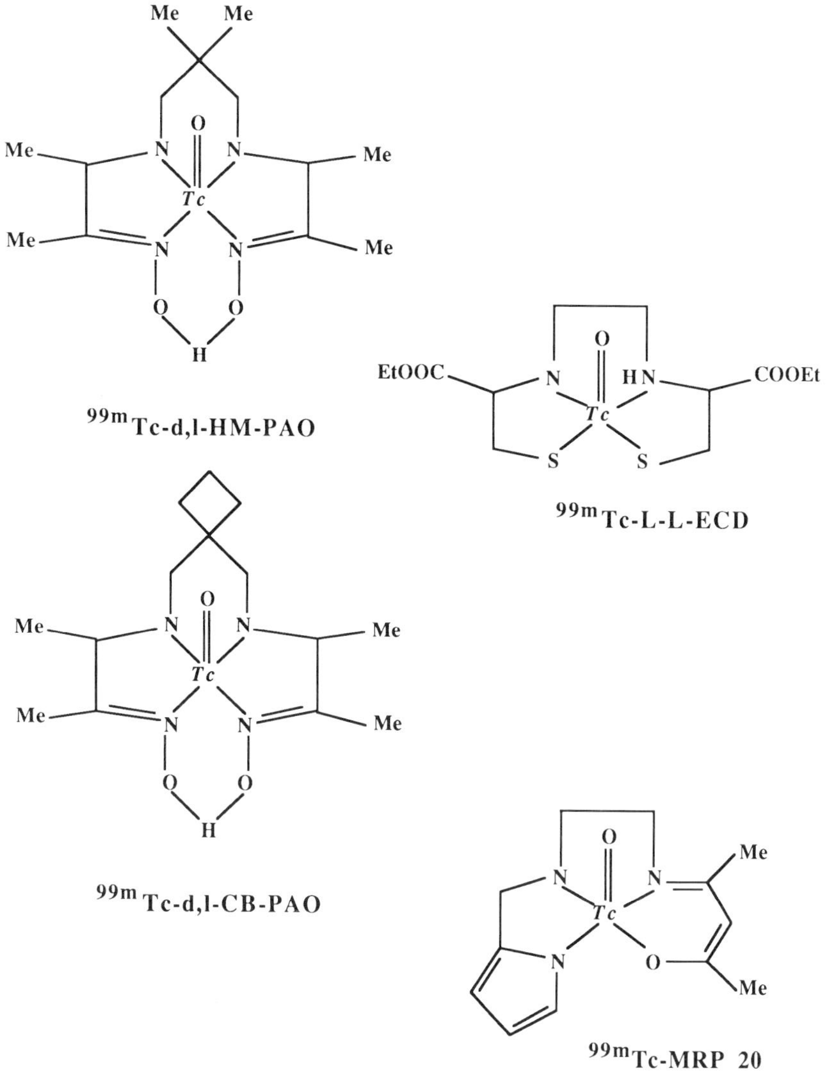

**Fig 5.** Chemical structures of HMPAO, CBPAO, ECD and MRP 20.

form neutral and lipophilic complexes with $^{99m}$Tc that are decomposed in vivo into more polar metabolites (Morgan et al. 1990).

$^{99m}$Tc-HMPAO (Amersham International) is the only compound approved for use in Europe and it is also approved by the FDA for use in the USA. The largest body of experience of clinical utility has been compiled with this compound, with extensive clinical work having been undertaken in the USA, Japan and Europe. Normal CBF SPET templates are being developed for this compound in various centres with ongoing comparative data with MRI and CT.

The main drawback of $^{99m}$Tc-HMPAO is the need for rapid administration of

Table 2. $^{99m}$Tc-labelled cerebral perfusion agents[a]

|  | $^{99m}$Tc-D,L,-HMPAO | $^{99m}$Tc-L,L-ethyl cysteinate dimer (ECD) | $^{99m}$Tc-(N-(2(1H pyrolylmethyl))N'-(4-pentene-3-one-2)) ethane 1,2 diamine)) (MRP-20) |
|---|---|---|---|
| Other names | $^{99m}$Tc-D,L, hexamethylpropylene amine oxime, $^{99m}$Tc-PAO, $^{99m}$Tc-exametazine | $^{99m}$Tc-ethylcysteinate dimer, $^{99m}$Tc-ethylene-dicysteine diethylester, $^{99m}$Tc-ECD |  |
|  | Ceretec | Neurolite | Neuroscint |
| Preparation | Kit, R.T. | Kit, R.T. | Kit, R.T. |
| Stability | 30 min | >6 h | ? |
| Activity | 1.11 GBq | 3.70 GBq | ? |
| Brain uptake at 1 h post-injection (% I.D.) | 6.05 | 5.2 | 5.2 |
| Redistribution | No | No | No |
| Retained species | Polar metabolite | Mono-ester | Hydrolysed metabolite |
| In blood (%), 1 h | 12.0 | 4.9 | 24 |
| In urine (%) after 24 h | 38 | 74 | 30 |
| Status | Approved | Phase III C.T. | Phase I C.T. |

[a]Origin of data: Costa et al. (1986); Sharp et al. (1986); Neirinckx et al. (1987); Holman et al. (1989); Léveillé et al. (1989); Bossuyt et al. (1990a,b, 1991); Walovitch et al. (1990).

Table 3. Dosimetry of $^{99m}$Tc-brain agents (mGy/740 MBq)[a]

|  | $^{99m}$Tc-D,L,-HMPAO | $^{99m}$Tc-L,L-ECD | $^{99m}$Tc-MRP 20 |
|---|---|---|---|
| Brain | 3.0 | 3.6 | 4.4 |
| Bladder wall[b] | 10.4 | 22.0 | 1.6 |
| Kidneys | 19.4 | 5.6 | 23.0 |
| Liver | 8.4 | 3.6 | 10.2 |
| Lungs | 1.8 | 1.4 | 11.8 |
| Intestines | — | — | 34.0 |
| – Small intestine | 22.0 | 7.0 | — |
| – Upper large intestine wall | 36.0 | 12.0 | — |
| – Lower large intestine wall | 15.6 | 9.6 | — |
| Bone marrow | 4.8 | 1.6 | 2.0 |

[a]Origin of data: Neirinckx et al. (1987); Holman et al. (1989); Bossuyt et al. (1990)
[b]2-h voiding

the compound after its reconstitution with $^{99m}$Tc. Once HMPAO is labelled, it is inherently unstable – the tracer decomposes rapidly with time into a mixed proportion of species with variable liposolubility. It must therefore be prepared rapidly in the hot laboratory and used on patients without delay.

Several methods have been described that improve the stability of HMPAO (Hung et al. 1989; Verbruggen 1990), of which the new cyclobutyl compound (CBPAO) is the most interesting. In this case a CB ring structure is used, resulting in a much greater amount of in vitro stability.

There are further differences in the behaviour of these compounds which relate to blood clearance, urinary excretion, dosimetry and washout from the brain. We have shown in earlier experiments that $^{99m}$Tc-ECD does wash out from the brain – this does not occur with HMPAO.

# Radiopharmaceuticals: Receptors

A neurotransmitter is a diffusible chemical that conveys information, usually regarding the state of membrane depolarization, from one neuron to another across a tiny gap called the synapse (Perry 1991).

As described in a recent article (Mazière and Mazière 1990), receptors represent large proteins or glycoproteins which, at the surface of the cell, have the ability to identify and bind, by weak non-covalent-type binding, specific compounds, often referred to as ligands. They also have the ability to pass on information to within the cell or to the surrounding milieu. They can therefore act as messengers that can regulate the level of excitation of the target cell, the amount of transmitter substance released from pre-synaptic terminals or even trigger post-synaptic events. More than 40 types of such messengers have already been identified (Iversen 1982).

In the nervous system, three categories of intercellular messengers can be defined: amino acids, monoamines and peptides. As stated by Bloom (1985), these tend to be present in quantities of micromole/milligram protein, nanomole/milligram protein and picomole/milligram protein.

These neuroreceptors are responsible for or take part in the regulation of many important biological and biochemical functions in the body, and in the brain in particular. These include the dopaminergic receptor systems (there are now at least three dopamine receptors being investigated, namely the D1,D2 and D3 receptors: Costa et al. 1990) where the neurotransmitter dopamine is stored in the pre-synaptic vesicles and released in order to act on its post-synaptic receptor sites, the opioid receptor system which is related to the mediation of pain, the benzodiazepine and GABA receptor systems, the serotonin receptor system, nicotinic and muscarinic receptors and so on.

As with antigens and monoclonal antibodies, receptors and ligands represent highly specific recognition systems. They can be successfully labelled with the radioactive tracer method and hence offer an entire new avenue for

Table 4. Neuroimaging and SPET neuroreceptor ligands

| Receptor | Ligand | Receptor | Ligand |
|---|---|---|---|
| M1,M2 | $^{123}$I-QNB<br>$^{123}$I-Dexetimide | BZ/GABA | $^{123}$I-Flumazenil |
| D2 | $^{123}$I-IBZM<br>$^{123}$U-2-Spiperone<br>$^{123}$I-iodolisuride | Serotonin $S_2$ | $^{123}$I-Ketanserin |
| D1 | $^{123}$I-SCH 23892<br>$^{123}$I-SCH 23390 | Opioid | $^{123}$I-Diprenorphine |
|  |  | Amines | $^{123}$I-IMP |

**Table 5.** In these tables, generally physiological agonists and synthetic antagonists are mentioned. An exception is made for the CBZ-GABAa receptor, at which both the physiological agonist for the GABAa receptor (GABA) and the hypothetical physiological agonist for the CBZ and PBZ receptor (DBI) are mentioned, as well as a synthetic BZ agonist. Another exception is made for the opiate receptors, for which besides the physiological agonists (enkephalins and endorphins) also some synthetic agonists are mentioned.
Adapted from N.P.L.G. Verhoeff (1991) Pharmacological Implications for Neuroreceptor Imaging. *European Journal of Nuclear Medicine* 18 (7) (In press).

## A. Acetylcholine

| Receptor | Second messenger | Agonist | Antagonist | Ligand (SPET) |
|---|---|---|---|---|
| M1 | PI, $Ca^{2+}$, cGMP | Acetylcholine | Pirenzepine | $^{123}$I-QNB[c] |
| M2 | cAMP (inhibits), $K^+$ | Acetylcholine | AFDX-116 | $^{123}$I-Dexetimide[b] |
| M3 | PI, $Ca^{2+}$, cGMP | Acetylcholine | HHSiD | |
| N | $Na^+$, $K^+$, $Cl^-$ | Acetylcholine | Alpha-BuTX | $^{125}$I-Nicotine[b] |
| | | | | $^{125}$I-DIP[b] |
| | | | | $^{125}$I-alpha-BuTX[a] |
| | | | | $^{125}$I-Dendrotoxin[a] |

## A. Acetylcholine (contd)

| Receptor | Ligand (PET) | Disease | Expectation |
|---|---|---|---|
| M1 | $^{11}$C-MQNB[b] | Alzheimer | −/= |
| M2 | $^{11}$C-TRB[c] | Huntington | − |
| M3 | $^{18}$F-DPET[b] | Chronic alcoholism | − |
| | $^{11}$C-DPET[b] | Alcohol abstinence | + |
| | | Barbiturate abstinence | + |
| | | Insecticides | − |
| N | $^{11}$C-Nicotine | Alzheimer | − |
| | | Smoking | + |

## B. Biogenic amines

| Receptor | Second messenger | Agonist | Antagonist | Ligand (SPET) |
|---|---|---|---|---|
| Alpha1 | PI, $Ca^{2+}$, cGMP | Noradrenaline | Prazosin | $^{125}$I-BE 2254[a] |
| | | | | $^{125}$I-HEAT[a] |
| | | | | $^{125}$I-Iodoazidoaryl-prazosin[a] |
| Beta1 | cAMP (stimulates) | Noradrenaline | Metoprolol | $^{123}$I-Prenalterol[b] |
| Beta2 | cAMP (stimulates) | Noradrenaline | ICI 118, 551 | $^{125}$I-ICYP[c] |
| | | | | $^{125}$I-IHYP[c] |
| | | | | $^{125}$I-IPIN[c] |
| D1 | cAMP (stimulates) | Dopamine | SCH 23390 | $^{123}$I-SCH 23982[b] |
| | | | | $^{123}$I-FISCH[b] |
| | | | | $^{123}$I-TISCH[b] |
| D2 | cAMP (inhibits), PI | Dopamine | Sulpiride | $^{123}$I-IBZM[c] |
| | | | | $^{123}$I-NCQ 298[b] |
| | | | | $^{123}$I-Epipride[c] |
| | | | | $^{123}$I-2-Spiperone[c] |
| | | | | $^{123}$I-ILIS[c] |
| | | | | $^{123}$I-IBF[b] |
| | | | | $^{131}$I-Iodo-tropapride[b] |
| | | | | $^{123}$I-IMD[b] |
| | | | | $^{123}$I-Haloperidol[a] |
| 5-HT1B | PI, $Ca^{2+}$ | Serotonin | Iodocyanopindolol | $^{125}$I-ICYP[a] |
| 5-HT1C | PI, $Ca^{2+}$ | Serotonin | MES | $^{125}$I-LSD[a] |
| 5-HT2 | cAMP (stimulates) | Serotonin | Ritanserin | $^{123}$I-2-Ketanserin[c] |
| | | | | $^{125}$I-DOI[a] |
| 5-HT3/1A | | Serotonin | OH-DPAT | $^{125}$I-Iodoethyl-spirotraxine[a] |
| H1 | PI, $Ca^{2+}$ | Histamine | Mepyramine | $^{125}$I-Iodobol-pyramine[b] |
| H2 | cAMP (stimulates) | Histamine | Cimetidine | |

Table 5 (continued)

## B. Biogenic amines (contd)

| Receptor | Ligand (PET) | Disease | Expectation |
|---|---|---|---|
| Beta1 | $^{11}$C-CGP 12177[a] | Cardiac decompensation | – |
| Beta2 | $^{11}$C-Carazolol[b] | Manic depressive psychosis | + |
| | $^{18}$F-FACarazolol[a] | Noradrenergic antidepressives | – |
| | $^{18}$F-FAPIN[c] | | |
| D1 | $^{11}$C-SCH 23390[c] | Extrapyramidal side effects with L-DOPA therapy in Parkinson | + |
| | $^{11}$C-SCH 39166[b] | Atypical antipsychotics | – |
| D2 | $^{11}$C-IBZM[b] | Tardive dyskinesia | + |
| | $^{18}$F-NCQ 115[b] | Typical antipsychotics | – |
| | $^{11}$C-Raclopride[c] | Withdrawal of antipsychotics | + |
| | $^{11}$C-NMSpiperone[c] | Huntington | – |
| | $^{18}$F-NFBSpiperone[a] | Multiple system atrophy | – |
| | $^{11}$C-NMBenperidol[b] | Parkinson "on" | + |
| | $^{11}$C-YM 09151-2[b] | Parkinson "off" | – |
| | $^{77}$Br-Spiperone[c] | | |
| | $^{18}$F-IBZM[b] | | |
| | $^{18}$F-FABZM[b] | | |
| 5-HT1B | | Manic depressive psychosis | + |
| 5-HT1C | | Manic depressive psychosis | + |
| 5-HT2 | $^{76}$Br-2-Ketanserin[a] | Manic depressive psychosis | + |
| | | Serotonergic antidepressives | – |
| | | Alzheimer | – |
| | | Anxiety | + |
| | | Alcoholism | – |
| | | Aggression | +/– |
| | | Suicidal ideation | +/– |
| | | Autism | +/– |
| 5-HT3/1A | $^{11}$C-MDL 72222[a] | Anxiety | + |
| | | Manic depressive psychosis | + |
| | | Serotonergic antidepressives | – |
| | | Alzheimer | – |
| | | Alcoholism | – |
| | | Aggression | +/– |
| | | Suicidal ideation | +/– |
| | | Autism | +/– |
| H1 | $^{11}$C-Pyrilamine[b] | Manic depressive psychosis | + |
| H2 | $^{11}$C-Ranitidine[a] | Heart failure | – |
| | | Epilepsy | + |

Table 5 continued overleaf

Table 5 (continued)

## C. Amino acids

| Receptor | Second messenger | Agonist | Antagonist | Ligand (SPET) |
|---|---|---|---|---|
| CBZ-GABAa | $Cl^-$ | GABA, DBI(?), Diazepam, Flunitrazepam | Bicuculline, Flumazenil | $^{123}$I-Iomazenil$^c$ $^{123}$I-2'-IDZ$^b$ $^{123}$I-G-018$^b$ |
| PBZ | | DBI(?) Diazepam | PK 11195 | $^{125}$I-PK 11195$^b$ |
| NMDA | | Glutamate | MK 801 | $^{125}$I-3-MK 801$^b$ |

## C. Amino acids (contd)

| Receptor | Ligand (PET) | Disease | Expectation |
|---|---|---|---|
| CBZ-GABAa | $^{11}$C-Flumazenil$^c$ $^{11}$C-NMDZ$^b$ $^{18}$F-FERO, $^{18}$F-FPRO$^b$ $^{11}$C-Alprazolam$^b$ | Lennox-Gastaut syndrome Temporal epilepsy Chronic alcoholism Alzheimer Anxiety disorder | − −/= − − −/= |
| PBZ | $^{11}$C-PK 11195$^c$ $^{18}$F-PK 14105$^b$ | Glioma | + |
| NMDA | $^{18}$F-13MMK 801$^b$ | Epilepsy Hypoxia | + +/− |

## D. Neuropeptides

| Receptor | Second messenger | Agonist | Antagonist | Ligand (SPET) |
|---|---|---|---|---|
| Delta, Kappa and Mu | cAMP (inhibits) | Enkephalins Dynorphine Endorphin | Mr 2266 Mr 2266 | |
| Mu | | Morphine | Naltrexone | |
| Sigma | | (+)SKF10047, LMWfraction | Mr 2266 | $^{123}$I-PIPAg$^b$, $^{123}$I-MIPAG$^b$ |
| Vasopressin | cAMP (stimulates) | Vasopressin | AVA | $^{125}$I-AVA$^b$ |
| Oxytocin | PI, $Ca^{2+}$ | Oxytocin | OTA | $^{125}$I-OTA$^b$ |
| Insulin | cAMP (inhibits), PI | Insulin | | $^{125}$I-Insulin$^a$ |
| Somatostatin | cAMP (inhibits) | Somatostatin | Octreotide | $^{123}$I-Tyr-3-octreotide$^c$ |
| Melatonin | cAMP (stimulates) | Melatonin | | $^{125}$I-IMEL$^b$ |
| Secretin | cAMP (stimulates) | Secretin | | $^{125}$I-Secretin$^a$ |
| VIP | cAMP (stimulates) | VIP | | $^{125}$I-VIP$^a$ |
| Substance P | PI, $Ca^{2+}$ | Substance P | | $^{125}$I-Substance P$^a$ |
| CCK | PI, $Ca^{2+}$ | Cholecystokinin | | |

## D. Neuropeptides (contd)

| Receptor | Ligand (PET) | Disease | Expectation |
|---|---|---|---|
| Delta, Kappa and Mu | $^{11}$C-Diprenorphine$^c$ $^{18}$F-NPDiprenorphine$^b$(?) $^{11}$C-Cyclofoxy$^b$ | Absence seizures | − |
| Mu | $^{11}$C-Carfentanyl$^c$ $^{11}$C-Ohmefentanyl$^a$ $^{11}$C-Buprenorphine$^a$ | Partial epilepsy | + |
| Sigma | $^{11}$C-MPAG$^2$ | Schizophrenia | + |
| Insulin | | Diabetes mellitus type II | − |
| Somatostatin | | Gastrinoma, carcinoid Pancreatic endocrine tumour Paraganglioma | + + + |
| Melatonin | | | |
| Secretin | | | |
| VIP | | | |
| Substance P | | | |
| CCK | $^{11}$C-MK 329 | Irritable bowel syndrome | + |

**Table 5** (*continued*)

**E. Steroids**

| Receptor | Second messenger | Agonist | Antagonist | Ligand (SPET) |
|---|---|---|---|---|
| MC Type I | DNA-mRNA | Aldosterone | Spironolactone | |
| GC Type II | DNA-mRNA | Cortisol | | |
| E2 | DNA-mRNA | Oestradiol | Tamoxifen | $^{123}$I-Z-17alpha-IV-oestradiol$^b$ $^{125}$I-16alpha-iodo-oestradiol$^b$ |
| T | DNA-mRNA | Testosterone | Cyproteronacetate | |

**E. Steroids (contd)**

| Receptor | Ligand (PET) | Disease | Expectation |
|---|---|---|---|
| MC Type I | $^{18}$F-RU 26752$^b$ | Conn | − |
| GC Type II | $^{18}$F-RU 28362$^b$ | Addison | + |
| | $^{18}$F-21-Deacyl-cortivazol$^b$ | Cushing | − |
| | $^{18}$F-RU-52461$^b$ | Chronic steroid therapy | − |
| E2 | $^{18}$F-16 alpha-FES$^c$ | Carcinoma breast | + |
| | $^{18}$F-Tamoxifen$^a$ | | |
| T | $^{18}$F-20-Mibolerone$^b$ | Prostate carcinoma | + |

**F. Purines**

| Receptor | Second messenger | Agonist | Antagonist | Ligand (SPET) |
|---|---|---|---|---|
| A1 | cAMP (inhibits) | Adenosine | PACPX | |

**F. Purines (contd)**

| Receptor | Ligand (PET) | Disease | Expectation |
|---|---|---|---|
| A1 | $^{18}$F-FMB-XCC$^a$ | Anxiety disorder | − |
| | $^{11}$C-CPT$^a$ | Epilepsy | − |
| | | Pain | + |
| | | Lesch-Nyhan syndrome | − |

a = tested in vitro in laboratory animals
b = tested in vivo in laboratory animals
c = tested in human subjects
+ = receptor density measured is expected to be increased
− = receptor density measured is expected to be decreased

the investigation of health and disease and the application of nuclear medicine.

Both SPET and PET are already actively engaged with this methodology. It is appropriate to pay homage to Crawley et al. (1983), who early on documented the potential of this with bromine-77 methyl-spiperone and SPET. In the same year, the group from Johns Hopkins with Wagner et al. (1983) published their PET study on the imaging of dopamine receptors in the human brain. Steady progress has been made with SPET and PET, and even the radiopharmaceutical industry is actively included now – a number of tracers are being made available for almost routine use in nuclear medicine.

There are many interesting issues to be solved. Concentrations of the neuroreceptors is always rather low ($10^{-12}$ mole/gram of brain tissue) the binding affinity between receptor and ligand is also very small ($10^{-6}$ M to $10^{-9}$ M) and very high specific activity concentration of label will have to be used (greater than a 1000 Ci/M) in order to prepare a neuroreceptor imaging agent successfully. The development of a number of highly sensitive imaging tomographs is not only timely but necessary if studies are to be carried out on significant numbers of patients.

Concentration or receptor density is difficult to measure; receptors may be up- or down-regulated and many different stimuli or events may give rise to a similar response of a specific receptor system.

Labelling of these neuroreceptor ligands has not been achieved so far with $^{99m}$Tc. This is also unlikely to occur in the near future. The radionuclide of choice is $^{123}$I, an isotope with an energy for imaging of 159 keV and a physical half-life of 13 h. The cost per unit of radioactivity is much higher for this radionuclide than for $^{99m}$Tc and its availability and geographical distribution are much more restricted.

The implications are clear. $^{123}$I-labelled neuroreceptor imaging is expensive, only available on a restricted basis and confined to a rather limited number of centres worldwide. Clinical research is, however, ongoing and progressing using a widening range of such tracers. The main neuroreceptor ligands being investigated by SPET are listed in Table 4. Table 5 provides for a more comprehensive list of ligands with a possible future (Verhoeff 1991).

# References

Baker JHL, Campbell JK, Houser OW, et al (1974) Computer assisted tomography of the head. An early evaluation. Mayo Clin Proc 49:17–27

Biersack HJ, Coenen HH, Stöcklin G, et al (1989) Imaging of brain tumours with L-3-[$^{123}$I]Iodomethyl tyrosine and SPECT. J Nucl Med 30:110–112

Black HL, Hawkins RA, Kim KT, et al (1989) Thallium-201 (SPECT): a quantitative technique to distinguish low grade from malignant brain tumours. J Neurosurg 71:342–346

Bloom FE (1985) Neurotransmitter diversity and its functional significance. J R Soc Med 78:189–192

Bossuyt A, Pirotte R, Chirico A, et al (1990a) Whole body dosimetry of Tc-99m-MRP 20: the result of a phase I clinical trial. Eur J Nucl Med 16:432

Bossuyt A, Pirotte R, Chirico A, et al (1990b) Tc-99m-MRP 20, a new brain perfusion agent suitable for SPECT imaging. Eur J Nucl Med 16:418

Bossuyt A, Pirotte R, Carroll MJ, et al (1991) Tc-99m-MRP 20, a new brain perfusion agent suitable for SPECT imaging. In: Schmidt HAE, van der Schoot JB (eds) Nuclear medicine. The state of the art of nuclear medicine in Europe. Schattauer, Stuttgart New York, pp 222–224

Bradbury MWB (1985) Transport across the cerebral endothelium. Circ Res 57:213–222

Carril JM, MacDonald AF, Dendy PP, et al (1979) Clinical scintigraphy: value of adding emission computed tomographic studies to conventional pertechnetate images (512 cases). J Nucl Med 20:1117–1123

Clark SEM, Harding K, Buxton TM (1990) The current cost of nuclear medicine. Nucl Med Commun 11:527–538

Costa DC, Ell PJ, Cullum ID, et al (1986) The in vivo distribution of 99Tcm-HM-PAO in normal man. Nucl Med Commun 7:647–658

Costa DC, Verhoeff NPLG, Cullum ID, et al (1990) In vivo characterisation of 3-iodo-6-methoxybenzamide 123-I in humans. Eur J Nucl Med 16:813–816

Crawley JCW, Smith T, Veall N, et al (1983) Dopamine receptors displayed in living human brain with $^{77}$Br-p-bromospiperone. Lancet I:975

Deland FH (1971) Scanning in cerebral vascular disease. Semin Nucl Med 1:31–40

Dempsey EW, Wislocki GB (1955) An electron microscopic study of the blood-brain barrier in the rat. J Biophys Biochem Cytol 1:245

Ell PJ, Deacon JM, Ducassou D, et al (1980) Emission and transmission brain tomography. BMJ 280:438–440

Ell PJ, Cullum I, Costa DC, et al (1985) A new regional cerebral blood flow mapping with Tc-99m-labelled compound. Lancet II:50–51
Fischer RJ, Miale A Jr (1972) Evaluation of cerebral vascular disease with radionuclide angiography. Stroke 3:1–9
Glasco JL, Currier RD, Goodrich JK, et al (1965) Brain scans at varied intervals following CVA. J Nucl Med 6:902–916
Gruber ML, Hochberg FH (1990) Editorial: systematic evaluation of primary brain tumours. J Nucl Med 31:969–971
Hill TC, Lovett RD, Zimmerman RE (1980) Quantification of Tc-99m glucoheptonate uptake in brain lesions with emission-computed tomography. In: Single photon emission computed tomography and other selected computer topics. Society of Nuclear Medicine, New York, pp 169–176
Holman BL, Hellman RS, Goldsmith SJ, et al (1989) Biodistribution, dosimetry and clinical evaluation of technetium-99m ethyl cysteinate dimer in normal subjects and in patients with chronic cerebral infarction. J Nucl Med 30:1018–1024
Hopkins GG, Kristensen KAB (1973) Rapid sequential scintiphotography in the radionuclide detection of subdural hematoma. J Nucl Med 14:288–290
Hounsfield GN (1973) Computerised transverse axial scanning (tomography): Part 1. Description of system. Br J Radiol 46:1016–1022
Hung JC, Volkert WA, Holmes RA (1989) Stabilization of technetium-99m-D,L-hexamethylpropyleneamine oxime (99mTc-D,L-HMPAO) using gentisic acid. Nucl Med Biol 16:675–680
Iversen LL (1982) Neurotransmitters and CNS disease. The Lancet II:914–918
Kaplan WD, Takronan T, Morris H, et al (1989) Thallium-201 brain tumour imaging: a comparative study with pathologic correlation. J Nucl Med 28:47–52
Kim KT, Black KL, Marciano D, et al (1990) Thallium-201 SPECT imaging of brain tumours: methods and results. J Nucl Med 31:965–969
Knapp WH, Von Kummaer R, Kübler W (1986) Imaging of cerebral blood flow-to-volume distribution using SPECT. J Nucl Med 27:465–470
Kung HF, Blau M (1980) Synthesis of selenium-75 labelled tertiary diamines: new brain imaging agents. J Med Chem 23:1127–1130
Léveillé J, Demonceau G, De Roo M, et al (1989) Characterization of technetium-99m-L, L-ECD for brain perfusion imaging, part 2. Biodistribution and brain imaging in humans. J Nucl Med 30:1902–1910
Libson K, Messa C, Kwiatkowski M et al (1989) $^{99m}$Tc-MRP-20. A new class of neutral complex with implications for brain scintigraphy. J Nucl All Sci 33:305–306
Maynard CD, Witcofski RL, Janeway R et al (1969) Radioisotopic arteriography as an adjunct to the brain scan. Radiology 92:908–912
Mazière B, Mazière M (1990) Where have we got with neuroreceptor mapping of the human brain? Eur J Nucl Med 16:817–835
Miller JW, Hess A (1958) The blood-brain barrier: an experimental study with vital dyes. Brain 81:248
Morgan GF, Thornback JR, Deblaton M et al (1990) Development of a novel class of lipophilic technetium complexes designed to mimic rCBF (abstract 131). Eur J Nucl Med 16:423
Mountz JM, Stafford-Schuck K, McKeeven PE, et al (1988) Thallium-201 tumour/cardiac ratio estimation of residual astrocytoma. J Neurosurg 68:705–709
Neirinckx RD, Canning LR, Piper IM, et al (1987) Technetium-99m, d, 1-HM-PAO: a new radiopharmaceutical for SPECT imaging of regional cerebral blood perfusion. J Nucl Med 18:191–202
Perry EK (1991) Neurotransmitters and diseases of the brain. Br J Hosp Med 45:73–83
Reese TS, Karnovski MJ (1968) Fine structural localisation of a blood-brain barrier to exogenous peroxidase. J Cell Biol 34:207
Rollo FD, Cavalieri RR, Born M, et al (1977) Comparative evaluation of $^{99m}$TcGH, $^{99m}$TcO$_4$ and $^{99m}$TcDTPA as brain imaging agents. Radiology 123:379–383
Ryerson TW, Spies SM, Singh NB, et al (1978) A quantitative clinical comparison of three $^{99m}$technetium labelled brain imaging radiopharmaceuticals. Radiology 127:429–432
Sharp FF, Smith FW, Gemmell HG, et al (1986) Technetium-99m-HM-PAO stereoisomers as potential agents for imaging regional cerebral blood flow: human volunteer studies. J Nucl Med 27:171–177
Siccardi AG, Buraggi GL, Natali PG, et al (1989) Technetium-99m-ECD: a new brain imaging agent: in vivo kinetics and biodistribution studies in normal human subjects. J Nucl Med 30:599–604

Uzler JM, Bennett LR, Mena I, et al (1975) Human CNS perfusion scanning with $^{123}$I-iodoantipyrine. Radiology 115:197–200

Van Nerom C, Bormans G, De Beukelaer C, et al (1990) Metabolism of 99mTc-ECD in organ homogenates of baboon. In: Schmidt HAE, Chambron PD (eds) Nuclear medicine. Quantitative analysis in imaging and function. Schattauer, Stuttgart New York, pp 87–89

Van Royen EA, De Bruine JF, Hill TC, et al (1987) Cerebral blood flow imaging with thallium-201 diethyldithiocarbamate SPECT. J Nucl Med 28:178–183

Verbruggen AM (1990) Radiopharmaceuticals: state of the art. Eur J Nucl Med 17:346–364

Verhoeff NPGL (1991) Pharmacological implications for neuroreceptor imaging. Eur J Nucl Med (in press)

Vyth A, Fennema PJ, Van der Schoot JB (1983) $^{201}$Tl-diethyldithiocarbamate: a possible radiopharmaceutical for brain imaging. Pharmacol Weekbl Sci 5:213–216

Wagner HN, Burner HD, Dannals RF, et al (1983) Imaging dopamine receptors in the human brain by PET. Science 221:1264–1266

Walovitch RC, Williams SJ, Lafrance ND (1990) Radiolabelled agents for SPECT imaging of brain perfusion. Nucl Med Biol 17:77–83

Waxman AD, Tanacescu D, Siemsen JK, et al (1976) Technetium-99m glucoheptonate as a brain scanning agent: critical comparison with pertechnetate. J Nucl Med 17:345–348

White DR, Muss HB, Cowan RJ (1976) Brain scanning in patients with advanced lung cancer. Clin Nucl Med 1:93–96

Chapter 3

# SPET Instrumentation: Characteristics and New Developments

## Introduction

According to the principles of emission imaging outlined in Chap. 1, a single-photon emission tomography (SPET) system must be able to detect gamma rays along a multitude of directions. How the transition is made from infinite sampling, as required by the mathematical theory (Radon 1917; Herman 1980), to finite sampling in practice is critical (Budinger 1980; Heller and Goodwin 1987). Therefore, the type and performance of different SPET systems are dependent on how the various directions are physically realized and how well they sample the region to be reconstructed.

Attempts to obtain tomographic cross sections of the body using radionuclides began early in 1963 (Kuhl and Edwards 1963). The SPET methodology that utilizes a single rotating gamma camera has gained a wide role in clinical practice and research, particularly in brain and heart studies (Kuhl et al. 1975; Hor 1988; Budinger 1990). This chapter provides an overview of SPET systems, the single rotating gamma camera being the most widely available. The emphasis is on recent developments that essentially achieve the simultaneous acquisition of data from more directions than previously possible. Basically, these systems consist of more than one collimated, position- and energy-sensitive detector, commonly gamma cameras. Within the framework provided by the above tomographic principle, several such systems are physically described.

An assessment of the performance of the GE/CGR Neurocam, the three-headed SPET instrument used throughout this book, is provided.

## The Tomographic Process

The principles of tomographic data acquisition using a single rotating gamma camera are illustrated in Fig. 1. The acquisition of a series of images from a number of positions (angles) around the patient identifies a set of equivalent strips or profiles, which are the data acquired from a transaxial section (slice)

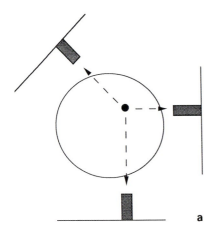

**Fig 1.** Demonstration of the principles of tomographic data acquisition. **a** Theoretical one dimensional (1-D) projections acquired by a position sensitive detector rotating around an object comprising a point source of radioactivity. **b** Real 2-D projections acquired by a gamma camera rotating around a patient's head.

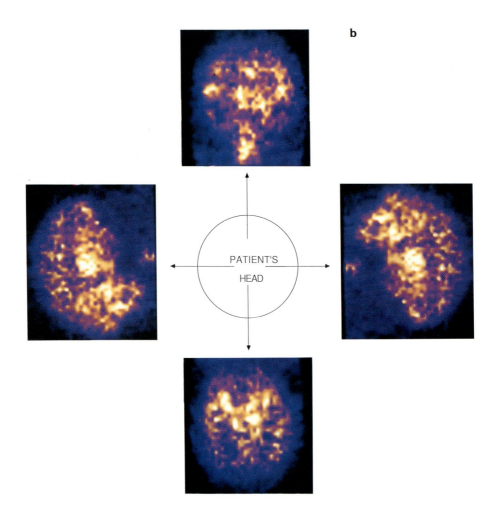

through the patient. Several of these sets of data can be acquired simultaneously using area detectors such as Anger gamma cameras. Single slice detectors provide data from just one section through the patient. The matrix size used for the projection images usually defines the maximum number of sets of data that are acquired simultaneously: a 64 × 64 matrix yields 64 sets (corresponding to 64 transaxial sections), a 128 × 128 matrix 128 sets, etc. Each element of image data within the strip, usually called a pixel, can be considered to represent the sum of activity along a line parallel to the hole direction in the collimator. For a parallel hole collimator this will be perpendicular to the detector and hence the axis of rotation. This condition is true in an ideal detector exhibiting infinite resolution and where attenuation and scatter are not present in the object being imaged. It is clear that none of these conditions apply in practice. The limitations thus imposed are discussed in later sections of this chapter.

For the ideal case, an exact solution exists for the reconstruction of a transaxial image from the projection profiles. The solution was first given at the beginning of this century (Radon 1917) and implementations have been used in tomographic imaging techniques in both radiology and nuclear medicine. Two methods of reconstruction have achieved considerable success (Herman 1980; Williams 1985): (a) filtered back-projection; (b) iterative reconstruction.

## Filtered Back-Projection

This is an analytical technique which, in the ideal case, would produce an exact solution to the reconstruction problem. If the data do not conform to the theoretical requirements, this process can be modified to yield acceptable results if the projection data are reasonably consistent.

The filtered back-projection process is illustrated in Fig. 2 and can be divided

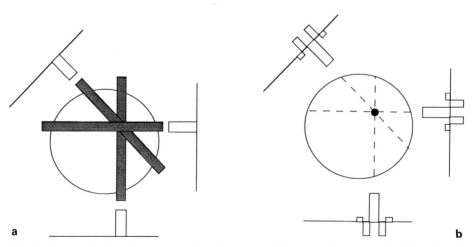

**Fig 2.** Demonstration of the principles of tomographic reconstruction using the filtered back-projection method. **a** Using the projection data of Fig. 1a, back-projection leads to the visualization of the point source by superposition. A star-like artifact is generated. **b** Filtering modifies the projection data so that after back-projection, the artifact is no longer evident.

into two parts, the first of which is back-projection, which can be seen as the inverse of the acquisition process. The pixel data, representing the sum along a line at a specified angle through the object, is reprojected onto the reconstruction image plane along the same line. The assumption made is that the original data were uniformly distributed throughout the object. This is the simplest and most fair assumption since the true distribution is unknown. When the process is repeated for all angles, one obtains a superposition of data which results in a blurred image. The blurring arises from the fact that each radioactive 'point' in the slice is reconstructed as a star-like distribution with rays corresponding to the back-projection angles. Where valid structures exist, there is a reinforcement due to the superposition of the back-projected data. However, the associated blurring defeats the purpose of the tomographic process, which is to increase image contrast. The second part of the reconstruction process is that of filtering. This can be subdivided into two components: the first is a filter to compensate for the blurring effect described above; the second is a filter to reduce the effect of inconsistencies in the data, particularly those due to statistical counting errors in the projection images. Modifications may be applied to seek to compensate for attenuation and scattering.

In order to understand the principles of filtering it is necessary to recognize that objects can be represented by a number of sinusoidal components of a specified amplitude and frequency, where frequency relates to the rate of change of the component. For example, an object that is essentially uniform has only zero (low) frequency components. Objects that exhibit variations in their properties in $X$ and $Y$ require the addition of higher frequency components to be correctly represented. A point object can be defined by the addition of components with frequencies ranging from zero to infinity. Given an object, these components are determined by a mathematical process called Fourier Transformation. The object is then said to be represented in Fourier or 'frequency space'.

The filter required to compensate for the blurring effect can be defined mathematically as a 'ramp' in frequency space. The zero frequency component remains unmodified and other frequencies are amplified in proportion to their frequency. Real data include statistical counting errors, which are present as high frequency components. Hence, the amplification properties of the ramp filter result in a dramatic increase in the noise present in the reconstructed image, usually resulting in an uninterpretable result. The second filter is used to reduce the noise. This requires the selection of a frequency value above which components added into the reconstructed image are rejected. These filters can be defined mathematically and govern the way in which the frequencies are modified. All require the selection of a 'cut-off' frequency that defines the frequency limit referred to above. In more conventional terms, this filter is a smoothing filter – the lower the cut-off frequency, the smoother the reconstructed image will appear. Clearly, filtering influences the achievable resolution in the reconstructed image (Fig. 3). There is no universally optimum filter; rather, the choice is dependent on the object to be reconstructed and the total number of counts detected (Gilland et al. 1990). The maximum (best) achievable resolution cannot be better than the system planar resolution.

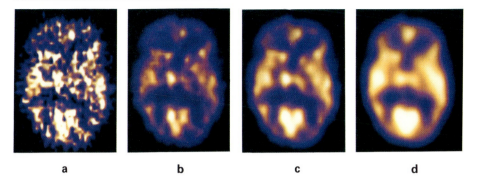

**Fig 3a–d.** The choice of filter and filter parameters affects image quality, both in terms of resolution and noise. This is illustrated in the following reconstructed images of the same slice: **a** Ramp filter. **b** Hanning cut-off frequency 1.3 cycles/cm. **c** Hanning cut-off frequency 1.0 cycles/cm. **d** Hanning cut-off frequency 0.7 cycles/cm.

## Iterative Reconstruction

This method is based upon the idea of repetitive projection – back-projection operations starting with an initial estimate of the unknown distribution. At each step, the projection data that would have been obtained from the current estimate of the distribution are calculated and compared to the measured projection data. The difference is used to modify the current estimate. This cyclic process is repeated until the differences between the calculated and measured projections are within predefined limits. The type and manner in which the modification is applied are mathematically specified and differ for different iterative techniques. In general, iterative techniques require considerably more computational power than the analytical filtered back-projection method. However, they offer advantages where the data are known to be incomplete or less consistent than required for the analytical solution. In addition, iterative techniques produce smoother images. Most techniques for handling errors caused by attenuation and scattering of photons within the body use iterative techniques.

# Factors That Influence Reconstructed Image Quality

The reconstructed image quality depends on several acquisition and processing parameters. Some are dependent on the system and patient (or phantom) and others are user-defined: intrinsic spatial resolution, geometric collimator resolution, scatter within the patient or phantom, energy resolution, energy window, radius of rotation, number of planar projections, pixel size of the projections, counts per pixel and total counts acquired, filtering of the projections, reconstruction algorithm, attenuation correction, reconstruction matrix size, post-reconstruction filtering.

## Spatial Resolution

The effects of intrinsic spatial resolution and collimator geometric resolution are characterized by the system planar resolution (expressed as full width at half maximum (FWHM) mm). The improved intrinsic spatial resolution assures better system resolution, although it is the collimator that mostly dictates the system resolution. Improved energy resolution enables the use of a narrower and asymmetric energy window, which leads to better scatter rejection and therefore better resolution and contrast. Since the system planar resolution deteriorates with distance from the collimator, the shorter the radius of rotation the better. Thus, the imaging detectors must be as close as possible to the patient during their orbit. Non-circular orbits have been introduced for this purpose.

A high-resolution parallel hole collimator and a smoother reconstruction filter have been found to yield better-quality images than a more sensitive (and therefore lower resolution) collimator and a sharper filter (Mueller et al. 1986; Kouris et al. 1990). New collimator designs introduced to improve SPET resolution include cast collimators, which can be made with more uniform hole construction than the lead-foil type; new designs for brain imaging include the long-bore parallel hole and converging-fan beam collimators, as well as astigmatic collimators, which converge in both planes with different lines of focus. Some of these improve both sensitivity and resolution compared to parallel hole collimators.

## Spatial and Angular Sampling

The number of planar projections (views) and the pixel size define the angular and spatial sampling, respectively. In accordance with the principle of tomography, the larger the number of directions along which information is obtained, the better. Mathematical theory demands that all (infinite) line integrals are known. However, in practice, both the angular sampling and the spatial sampling are finite. The angular sampling interval is commonly 3–5°. The pixel size of the planar projections depends on the field of view and the matrix size; it is commonly in the range 3–7 mm.

## Partial Volume Effect

Spatial resolution, together with contrast and statistical noise, governs lesion detectability. If the resolution expressed as FWHM is not small enough relative to the volume of a lesion or other structure of interest (e.g. putamen), the reconstructed anatomical representation will not correspond to the true physical extent, and the reconstructed activity concentration will be underestimated. This is referred to as the partial volume effect and is due to inadequate sampling. As a general rule, a structure of interest can be reconstructed adequately if its size (length, thickness or diameter) is greater than $2 \times$ FWHM. Thus, the extent of the partial volume problem is reduced as resolution improves. Contrast is then also improved.

## Scattering Problem

There must be a correspondence between the direction of emission of a gamma ray and the point of its detection. It follows that if the gamma ray undergoes inelastic scattering and therefore loses energy and changes direction, the correspondence is lost and its detection will provide wrong directional information. The net effect is a loss in contrast. Ideally such a gamma ray should not be utilized for image formation and should therefore be rejected.

Unfortunately, although the energy resolution capability of modern cameras has improved, it is not good enough to reject the majority of scattered gamma rays on account of their lower energy except those that have scattered by a large angle; for $^{99m}$Tc this angle is equal to 53° if a symmetric 20% energy window is used. However, recent developments in on-line energy corrections allow the use of narrower photopeak windows, as well as asymmetric energy windows. Offpeak energy windows have demonstrated significant improvements in contrast. Our experience with the GE/CGR Neurocam confirms that the use of a 17% energy window and a 3% asymmetric shift to the higher energy side of the peak does improve contrast without an appreciable loss in sensitivity.

Scatter compensation techniques for SPET have been reviewed by Jaszczak et al. (1985). The most common one (Jaszczak et al. 1984) utilizes a dual-energy window, the photopeak window and the scatter window, so that two sets of projections are acquired simultaneously. Under the assumption that the scatter window data are correlated to the scattered events detected within the photopeak window, a proportion specified by a factor 'k' of the scatter window data is subtracted from the photopeak data either prior to or after image reconstruction. Although improvements in image quality and quantification have been reported (Jaszczak et al. 1984; Koral et al. 1990), scatter compensation techniques are still under development and not widely used in practice.

## Attenuation Problem

Whether a gamma ray undergoes scattering or absorption somewhere along its path, the information it carries about the strength of the radioactive concentration along the direction of emission is lost; the number of detected gamma rays along this direction would not be proportional to the radioactive concentration along the line. Because of the exponential dependence of these interactions, gamma rays emanating from deeper regions would suffer greater scattering and attenuation than from superficial regions, and the reconstructed activity concentrations would therefore be underestimated; typically, this leads to the outer rim of a reconstructed slice appearing brighter than it should.

In order for SPET to yield quantitative information on the distribution of activity, attenuation correction must be performed. Most conventional methods assume a uniform attenuation coefficient within the boundary of each slice (Chang 1978). This assumption is not unreasonable for the head (except for the skull), but these methods are totally inadequate for the chest and abdomen. The accurate solution of the attenuation problem requires accurate knowledge of the map of attenuation coefficients at the energy of the radionuclide used. Different approaches depend on how the map is obtained: (a) separate transmission scan using the same radionuclide as for the emission study (Malko et al. 1986); (b) simultaneous transmission scan using a lower energy source (Bailey et al. 1987); (c) previous X-ray CT scan (Fleming 1989). In practice, none of these methods is routinely applied, but the availability of multiheaded systems with their improved sensitivity may induce renewed interest for further developments, particularly with methods a and b.

## SPET Principles: Quality Control

The quality control (QC) procedures for SPET systems must be regarded as an extension to standard gamma-camera QC procedures, as detailed in a report by NEMA, the National Electrical Manufacturers' Association (NEMA 1986). SPET places more stringent requirements on the performance of the detectors than planar imaging. However, the SPET performance can be directly related to the planar imaging performance, especially with regard to resolution and sensitivity.

The quality-control procedures specific for SPET derive from the primary assumptions of the tomographic process. These can be summarized as follows:

1. The gamma camera/computer system has a uniform response to incident radiation. This not only implies a uniform sensitivity across the face of the detector but also that the energy and spatial resolutions are uniform throughout the field of view (FOV). Underlying these are the requirements for a uniform energy and spatial response, giving a correspondence between input and output energy and positional signals.

2. The reconstruction process maintains a 1:1 correspondence with the acquisition process and, in particular, the back-projection angle coincides with the acquisition angle and the back-projection centre of rotation coincides with the acquisition centre.

3. These requirements remain true regardless of the rotational position of the detector.

4. There is a direct correspondence between all detectors in a multiheaded system.

In order to ensure the adequate performance of a SPET system, a number of requirements must be met. Firstly, the detectors must have appropriate correction techniques for energy and spatial response. These are often called energy correction and linearity correction and may be calibrated by the manufacturer or the user, depending on system type. They seek to address the question of linearity of response with respect to energy and position and also act as part of the optimization of energy response. Secondly, the collimator often proves to be the weakest link in the imaging process. As has already been stated, it defines the relationship between the object and the image. Imperfections in collimator construction, particularly in regard to hole direction, result in distortions that can all too readily degrade image quality. Thirdly, the gantry and its subsequent installation are critical in maintaining the correspondence between the acquisition and reconstruction processes.

A detailed discussion of the acceptance procedures required for SPET systems is beyond the scope of this book and the reader is referred to a report by the AAPM, the American Association of Physicists in Medicine (AAPM 1987). Given the validity of the energy and linearity corrections, routine quality assurance can be simplified to calibrations for non-uniform sensitivity of response and identification of the mechanical centre of rotation to the reconstruction process. The latter may also provide a very powerful tool to confirm the integrity of the gantry system and the acquisition process.

A non-uniform response may lead to errors in the reconstructed image, which appear as concentric circles about the centre of rotation. Their magnitude will be dependent on the magnitude and shape of the error in the projection image and also on the position of that error in relation to the centre of rotation. Where the response of the detector varies rapidly, the errors will be larger and those closest to the centre of rotation will yield the largest amplitude of error in the reconstructed image. These problems are addressed by the acquisition of an image from a uniform source of activity from which multiplicative correction factors are obtained to correct the projection data post-acquisition or during the reconstruction process. Guidelines for the acquisition of these corrections are that the source and image data should have errors less than $\pm 1\%$ of the mean, representing a calibration image containing more than 10,000 counts/pixel. The correction image should be obtained with the same radionuclide as that used in patient studies, with the same pulse height analyser settings and with the same collimator. Other considerations such as the inclusion of a scatter component in the uniform activity source may also be needed (Lassen 1980).

The second and third requirements can be addressed together by considering their result, which is the incorrect alignment of projections. Such errors result in a gradual and often imperceptible degradation in resolution and contrast in the reconstructed images. A test of the system integrity and the identification of the position of the projection of the centre of rotation in the projection images can be obtained from a SPET acquisition of a point source. The source should be located approximately 10–15 cm away from the mechanical centre of rotation. Subsequent to the acquisition, the X and Y coordinates of the point source are derived from each projection image. If the system is observing a plane in space, then the Y coordinate will remain constant and the X coordinates should assume the characteristics of a sine wave. By subtracting the best fit sinusoid from these data, the residuals should be a horizontal line whose Y intercept defines the pixel value in the projection images corresponding to the mechanical centre of rotation. This value is used in the reconstruction process to align the projection images. Some systems identify multiple values for each acquisition angle, which will only be necessary if the criterion above is not met. An example of a typical output from a correctly functioning detection system is shown in Figure 4. Where the criteria above are not met, these usually indicate that the detector is not being maintained parallel to the rotation axis during acquisition or that the rotation increments are not equal. The causes of these effects are multiple and system-dependent.

Guidelines for this calibration and QC procedure are that the source must be as small as possible and that the result should be compared for each collimator to be used for patient studies, for each mode of acquisition (circular and patient

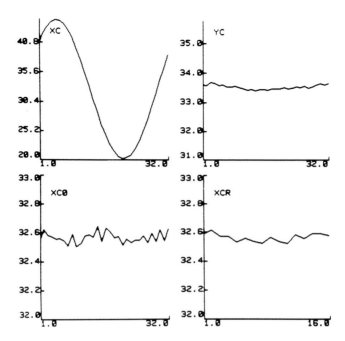

**Fig 4.** Results of a QC procedure for determination of the centre of rotation of a well functioning SPET system.

body contouring) and for both directions of rotation. Measurements should also be made at several positions along the Y axis (the patient axis) of the camera to verify that the same value is obtained at all positions. Similarly, where multidetector systems are used, similar values must be obtained for all detectors unless multiple correction files are used in the system. In general, a value derived from one measurement position on the detector face is applied to all other positions. A more detailed examination to determine the uniqueness of the calibration value should be performed at least on installation. Given the above calibration procedure, any variations in the centre of rotation value with angle should be less than 1–1.5 mm and similarly for the variations between detectors in the X and Y directions.

The frequency of these calibration procedures is system-dependent. Modern gantry systems show a level of stability, which means that tests of mechanical alignment can be performed on a monthly basis. The uniformity correction is dependent on detector stability and typically should be performed or at least assessed on a weekly basis. It may be necessary to augment these procedures with a daily quality-assurance measurement utilizing a tomographic three-dimensional phantom. The reconstructed images may then be inspected visually, but it is recommended that some form of quantification be used, with a comparison against established action thresholds to ensure an adequate performance of the entire system. Measures of tomographic uniformity and tomographic resolution are typical parameters, although statistical comparisons with calibration images may also prove useful.

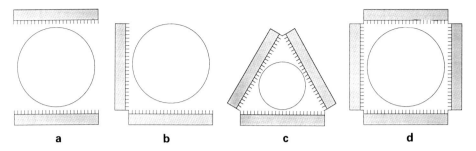

**Fig 5.** Possible geometric configurations of multi-headed SPET camera systems. **a** Two opposed cameras. **b** Two cameras at right angles. **c** Three cameras forming a triangle. **d** Four cameras forming a square.

## Multidetector/Multiheaded SPET

The realization that any improvements in resolution necessitate a loss in sensitivity (i.e. a further reduction in the fraction of the emitted gamma rays contributing to the imaging process) has led to the development of SPET systems with more than one gamma camera or with multiple detectors surrounding the patient's head or body. Figure 5 illustrates a number of possible detector configurations.

The increasing tendency towards the introduction of these systems has constituted a major advance because it has resulted in a significant increase in sensitivity. The gain factors that can be achieved are fundamentally dependent on the detector configuration chosen and the use of either 180° or 360° acquisition protocols. Table 1 indicates the relative scanning times for possible Anger gamma camera configurations. Figures are given for 180° and 360° protocols with data normalized to the time for a single detector. It is assumed that the detector characteristics are the same in all cases and any gains which may ensue from factors such as collimator type are ignored. The table does not consider non-Anger-type detectors.

Commercial manufacturers already offering multidetector systems are listed alphabetically in Table 2. It can be seen that there is little consensus as to the optimum detector configuration for a general purpose device; rather, the configuration is being chosen for a particular application or mix of applications.

The design goal of the new multiheaded instruments is to acquire data from

**Table 1.** Relative imaging times for different Anger gamma camera configurations

| Detectors | 180° | 360° |
|---|---|---|
| 1 Single | 1.0 | 1.0 |
| 2 Opposed | 1.0 | 0.5 |
| 2 Right angles | 0.5 | 0.5 |
| 3 Triangular | 0.67 | 0.33 |
| 4 Square | 0.5 | 0.25 |

Table 2. Commercial multidetector SPET systems

| Company | Model | No. of cameras or detectors | Organ |
| --- | --- | --- | --- |
| Adac | Genesys | 2 | Brain/body |
| DSI | Aspect | Annular | Brain |
| GE | ? | 2? | Brain/body |
| GE/CGR | Neurocam | 3 | Brain |
| Hitachi | SPECT 2000 | 4 | Brain |
| Medimatic | Tomomatic | 4 × 16 | Brain |
| Picker | PRISM | 3 | Brain/body |
| Shimadzu | Set-031 | 3 rings | Brain |
| Siemens | Multispect | 3 | Brain/body |
| SME | 810 | 12 | Brain |
| Toshiba | GCA-9300A | 3 | Brain/body |
| Trionix | Triad | 3 | Brain/body |

three dimensions with isotropic sampling and with high sensitivity. Volumetric imaging enables the study of an entire organ simultaneously rather than a single slice at a time as with single slice machines. Isotropic sampling ensures equal resolution in transverse, sagittal and coronal slices. Some of the increased sensitivity due to the detector configuration chosen can be sacrificed in pursuing higher resolution and hence reduced partial volume effects, better contrast and better quantitative accuracy.

High sensitivity also enables the use of radiopharmaceuticals the distribution of which changes with time, reflecting function or metabolism. With these multiheaded systems volumetric dynamic SPET is now possible. Previously this was only possible with high-sensitivity single-slice machines such as the Medimatic $^{133}$Xe scanner or the SME 810 (Lassen et al. 1978; Stoddart and Stoddart 1979).

In general, the gain in sensitivity can be exploited for optimizing the protocols according to which SPET procedures are performed. Depending on the aim of the clinical or research study in question, one can modify the parameters to produce either exquisite image quality better than achievable with a single conventional gamma camera, or the same image quality but with the data acquisition time significantly reduced, or reduce the administered dose to the patient. The pertinent parameters include the amount of administered radiopharmaceutical, collimator choice and total data-acquisition time.

The GE/CGR Neurocam system is one of the recent additions to the growing range of detector configurations available commercially. The design and performance of this device are described in the following section. A number of other systems are described in a later section to illustrate how the possible configurations outlined above have been implemented.

# GE/CGR Neurocam

The GE/CGR Neurocam comprises three Anger-type gamma cameras in a rotating gantry (Fig. 6). The cameras are rigidly fixed in the gantry, assuring

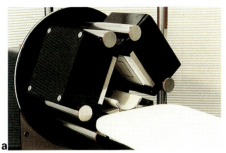 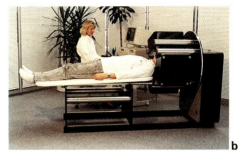

**Fig 6.** The GE/CGR Neurocam, a brain-dedicated SPET system, comprises three cameras. **a** The three cameras forming a triangular aperture for the patient's head. **b** The entire system has minimum demands on space.

mechanical stability. The front faces of the cameras form an almost equilateral triangular aperture within which the patient's head is positioned. The size of the aperture is constant; it is large enough to accommodate most adult heads but small enough to ensure close proximity imaging and hence better resolution; the radius of rotation is 11 cm. Each camera has 27 photomultiplier tubes (PMTs) coupled to a 6.5-mm-thick NaI(Tl) crystal with adequate shielding for gamma rays of energy up to 170 keV. The field of view is 20.0 cm × 17.6 cm. Unlike single-headed machines, patient positioning is easily and reproducibly done. The height of the headrest is fixed with respect to the gantry. The imaging table locks into place when pushed into the aperture. Collimators are light and easily handled. Data acquisition is controlled by an IBM-compatible personal computer. Data are energy-corrected on-line; linearity and uniformity corrections are made off-line for each planar image; centre of rotation corrections are made prior to tomographic reconstruction. Processing is performed on a GE Star 3000 computer after data transfer.

The various Neurocam corrections necessary for artefact-free SPET imaging remain valid sufficiently long, so that their updates do not constitute a burden to the patient load. We recommend that the centre of rotation offset values, the tuning values of the photomultiplier tubes (PMTs) and the energy (E)-corrections be updated weekly. Frequent acquisition of the uniformity corrections, as recommended for single rotating gamma cameras (weekly updates), is impractical for three-headed cameras because of time, cost and phantom considerations for each of the different radionuclides. The linearity corrections have remained valid since installation (at least 9 months). Switching from one radionuclide to another is quickly and efficiently done. Upon executing the required acquisition protocol, the appropriate PMT tuning values and E-corrections are loaded instantly and the window is well peaked on each camera.

## Physical Assessment of the GE/CGR Neurocam

### *Sensitivity*

The planar point source sensitivity of the Neurocam and the single-headed GE

400XCT camera was measured using a $^{99m}$Tc point source in air at 10 cm from the collimator. Values for different collimators are presented in Table 3.

The tomographic volume sensitivity of the Neurocam and the single-headed GE 400XCT camera was measured using a 20 cm diameter cylinder uniformly filled with $^{99m}$Tc; the length of the cylinder was greater than the FOV. The Neurocam sensitivities are 30.0 and 50.7 kcps/MBq/ml/cm for the HR and GP collimators, respectively. For comparison, the sensitivity of the single-headed GE 400XCT camera with GP collimator is 12.8 kcps/MBq/ml/cm, a factor of 3–4 less sensitive. Further results and comparison with another tomographic system, the SME 810 (see below), are presented in Table 3.

**Table 3.** Comparison of planar and tomographic sensitivity for the GE/CGR Neurocam, a single rotating gamma camera and the SME 810

*Planar sensitivity* (cpm/µCi) at 10 cm in air

| System | Collimator/window/offset | Planar sensitivity |
| --- | --- | --- |
| Neurocam | GP 140 keV 20%, 0% | 288 × 3 cpm/µCi |
|  | GP 140 keV 20%, 3% | 274 × 3 |
|  | HR 140 keV 20%, 0% | 167 × 3 |
|  | HR 140 keV 20%, 3% | 161 × 3 |
| GE 400XCT | HR 140 keV 20%, 0% | 183 |
|  | HR 140 keV 20%, 3% | 177 |

*Tomographic sensitivity*

| System | Collimator/window offset | Tomographic sensitivity |
| --- | --- | --- |
| GE/CGR Neurocam | GP 140 keV 20%, 0% | 50.7 kcps/MBq/ml/cm |
|  | GP 140 keV 20%, 3% | 47.4 kcps/MBq/ml/cm |
|  | HR 140 keV 20%, 0% | 30.0 kcps/MBq/ml/cm |
| GE 400XCT | GP 140 keV 20%, 0% | 12.8 kcps/MBq/ml/cm |
|  | GP 140 keV 20%, 3% | 11.1 kcps/MBq/ml/cm |
| SME 810 | Med Res 140 keV 20%, 0% | 315 kcps/MBq/ml/slice |
|  | Med Res 115–170 keV | 467 kcps/MBq/ml/slice |

## Resolution

The system planar resolution of the Neurocam and the single-headed GE 400XCT camera were measured using $^{99m}$Tc line sources. Table 4 provides a comparison of different collimators.

The tomographic spatial resolution of the Neurocam was evaluated using $^{99m}$Tc, $^{201}$Tl and $^{123}$I point and line sources. The SPET data acquisition parameters were: 128 projections 128 × 128 matrix, corresponding to a pixel size of 2.0 mm; reconstructions were performed using the Ramp filter. The reconstructed spatial resolution is isotropic in the three orthogonal planes: transaxial, sagittal and coronal. The full width at half maximum (FWHM) resolution in air at the centre of the field of view is 9.2 mm with the HR collimators. In water, it is 9.8 mm at the centre and 8.9 mm at 8 cm from the centre of the field of view. The Neurocam resolution is better than that of the single-headed GE 400XCT camera (Table 4). It is expected that the tomographic

**Table 4.** Comparison of system planar and reconstructed resolution of the GE/CGR Neurocam and a single-headed gamma camera

*System planar resolution* (FWHM mm) at 10 cm in air

|    | GE/CGR Neurocam | GE 400XCT |
|----|-----------------|-----------|
| HR | 8.1             | 8.1       |
| GP | 9.7             | 10.2      |
| HS |                 | 14.1      |

*Reconstructed resolution* (FWHM mm) in air at centre of FOV

|    | GE/CGR Neurocam | GE 400XCT         |
|----|-----------------|-------------------|
| HR | 9.2             | 13.5 (17 cm radius) |
| GP | 10.9            |                   |

resolution will improve further (by about 1–2 mm FWHM) with the forthcoming ultrahigh resolution (UHR) collimators.

## Data Sampling

Comparisons between 64 and 128 views, as well as between 64 × 64 and 128 × 128 matrix size, were performed with phantoms, volunteers and patients. There was an appreciable difference between 64 and 128 views of the brain, with 128 views yielding better images. However, 96 views may be sufficient and may lead to a reduction of data acquisition time and/or dose to the patient. There is an improvement in resolution and contrast if the 128 × 128 matrix is used, provided that attention is paid to noise due to counting statistics.

## Acquisition Protocols

Capitalizing on the increased sensitivity, the HR collimators are used for all studies with $^{99m}$Tc-HMPAO except where the patient is restless and the data acquisition time must be short. With such patients, a SPET study would not have been possible with a single rotating camera. The data acquisition parameters were: 64 or 128 projections, 64 × 64 or 128 × 128 matrix, 5–40 s per projection. Since at each step during the rotation, three projections are acquired simultaneously, the total acquisition time for a typical $^{99m}$Tc-HMPAO study with 128 projections and 20 s per projection takes about 14 min. Examples of the imaging protocols used and the resulting total counts and total acquisition times are listed in Table 5. The GP collimators are used for the $^{123}$I-IBZM studies because of the lower count rate. A dynamic $^{123}$I-IBZM study comprises 12 sequential tomographic scans at 10-min intervals, starting at 1 min post-injection. The acquisition parameters are: GP collimators, 64 views, 64 × 64 matrix, 15 s per view (i.e. 6 min total time per scan). Following the 12th scan a further dataset is acquired under the same conditions, except that the time per view is 60 s.

**Table 5.** Acquisition protocols for $^{99m}$Tc-HMPAO SPET using a single rotating gamma camera and the GE/CGR Neurocam

| Parameter | GE 400XCT | GE/CGR Neurocam | |
|---|---|---|---|
| Collimators | HR | HR | GP |
| No. of views | 64 | 128 | 128 |
| Matrix size | 128 | 64 | 64 |
| Pixel size (mm) | 3.2 | 4.0 | 4.0 |
| Time per view (s) | 30–40 | 20 | 15 |
| Total time (min) | 35–45 | 15 | 11 |
| Counts per view (kcnts) | 50 | 35 | 50 |
| Total counts (kcnts) | 3200 | 4480 | 6400 |

## Reconstruction Protocol

Transaxial tomographic reconstruction is performed using the filtered back-projection method. The projection data are prefiltered using the Hanning filter with cut-off frequency in the range 0.8–1.2 cycles/cm, depending on the total number of counts (higher for more counts). Back-projection is done using the Ramp filter. The attenuation correction procedure assumes a uniform linear attenuation coefficient of 0.12 cm$^{-1}$. Horizontal slices parallel to the OM-line, as well as sagittal and coronal slices, are generated from the transaxial dataset.

# Review of Other SPET Systems

There follows a brief description of some other commercial systems. Each description contains details of the detector sizes and configuration and whether they are capable of multiple or single slice acquisitions. Performance specifications have been included only where we have undertaken the measurements.

## Osaka/Hitachi SPECT 2000

The 4-headed Osaka/Hitachi SPECT 2000 is a brain-dedicated instrument (Kimura et al. 1990). It utilizes four compact gamma cameras rigidly fixed in a square arrangement that can be rotated at up to 6 rpm, permitting rapid dynamic SPET studies. Both step-and-shoot and continuous rotation modes are possible. Each camera comprises a NaI(Tl) crystal of thickness 9.0 mm coupled to 30 square PMTs in a 6 × 5 array. The distance between the collimator surfaces of opposed detectors is 26 cm. Hence the radius of rotation is 13 cm compared to 11 cm for the GE/CGR Neurocam. The field of view is 22.0 × 17.0 cm, similar to that of the Neurocam.

## ASPECT (DSI)

The annular single-crystal brain camera (ASPECT) consists of a stationary annular NaI(Tl) crystal and a rotating collimator system (Genna and Smith 1988; Holman et al. 1990). The FOV is 21.4 cm diameter by 10.7 cm in the axial direction. The internal diameter of the crystal is 31 cm and its thickness 8 mm. It is viewed by 63 PMTs arranged in three rings. Each PMT output is digitized so that all subsequent processing (including position computation, linearity and energy corrections) are digitally performed. The concentric collimator system comprises three parallel hole collimators viewing the head from three angles simultaneously. Collimator hole size is 1 mm, septal thickness 0.18 mm and length 2.4 cm. For comparison, the corresponding dimensions of the GE/CGR Neurocam HR collimators are 1.4 mm, 0.2 mm and 3.15 cm.

## Shimadzu Headtome SET-031

The Shimadzu Headtome SET-031 is a ring-type SPET system dedicated to the brain (Higashi et al. 1985). It comprises three rings of diameter 42 cm with 64 NaI(Tl) detectors each.

## SME 810

The SME Strickman Medical Equipment 810 is another brain-dedicated system, but it only scans one slice at a time (Stoddart and Stoddart 1979). Its principles of data acquisition and image reconstruction differ from those of the other systems described. It comprises 12 large (5 × 8 × 1 inches) NaI(Tl) detectors, 30° apart around a circle. Each detector is fitted with a point-focused collimator, which collects those photons that happen to travel towards the rectangular area of the detector along a set of lines traversing the focal point. Thus, a single measurement gives the number of counts detected over a solid angle with the focal point as the apex. During the scanning of one slice, each detector moves as a rectilinear scanner used to, so that the focal point raster scans through half the FOV; the opposing detector scans the other half simultaneously. During the scanning process, each detector takes 128 measurements along each line for 6 or 9 lines. The reconstructed spatial resolution measured using the high resolution collimators at our institution is 8.1 mm at the centre and 8.7 mm FWHM at 8 cm from the centre. This instrument is associated with high sensitivity (Table 3) but a significant fraction of the counts of each measurement are originating from slices other than the one being scanned. A reconstruction algorithm that deals with this problem is necessary (Moore and Mueller 1986).

## Toshiba GCA-9300A

In order to accommodate the body, three-headed systems such as the Toshiba GCA-9300A have been designed with a mechanically adjustable triangular aperture size. Bigger cameras are employed to allow body SPET data collection and hence the smallest triangle that can be achieved for imaging the brain is greater than that of the GE/CGR Neurocam. Although with parallel-hole collimators this leads to a degradation of spatial resolution, the use of fan beam collimators can offset the loss (Jaszczak et al. 1979; Tsui et al. 1986).

The Toshiba GCA-9300A comprises three rectangular gamma cameras with a 41 × 21 cm FOV (Ichihara 1990; Ichihara et al. 1990; Matsuda et al. 1990). Both parallel and fan beam collimators are available. Of particular interest are the low energy fan beam collimators used for the head (FOV is 21 × 22 cm diameter): (a) super-high resolution (SHR) made of lead; (b) ultra-high resolution (UHR) made of tungsten.

## Trionix TRIAD

The Trionix TRIAD system comprises three rectangular detectors arranged as a triangle within a closed ring-type gantry (Lim et al. 1985, 1986). The detectors can be moved radially to permit both high-resolution brain and body studies. Each detector utilizes 49 photomultiplier tubes with a useful field of view of 40 × 20 cm.

## Picker PRISM

As for the Triad, the PRISM system comprises three rectangular detectors, each with 49 photomultiplier tubes. The detectors are in a triangular configuration with radial motion allowed to provide for both brain and body imaging. The detectors are mounted in an open ring configuration rather than within a tunnel gantry. The useful field of view with parallel-hole collimators is 40 × 24 cm. This is reduced to 30 × 24 cm when fan beam collimators are employed. Collimators are available for a wide range of energies up to 400 keV.

# Discussion

Multidetector or multiheaded SPET systems primarily offer a substantial increase in sensitivity compared to a single rotating gamma. The triangular arrangement also offers the advantage that the cameras can be positioned relatively close to the patient's head or body.

Collimator choice is one of the most important factors that determine image quality in nuclear medicine (Sorenson and Phelps 1987). In spite of recommendations to use the high-resolution collimator in SPET (Keyes et al. 1990), many centres with single rotating gamma cameras continue to use the general purpose (and some the high sensitivity) collimator, presumably because they consider the sensitivity to be of paramount importance. While it is generally true that a compromise between resolution and sensitivity is necessary, we suggest that in reaching such a compromise for SPET, the resolution improvement be given a greater weight than the accompanying loss in sensitivity.

With the advent of multiheaded cameras and the consequential gain in sensitivity, the loss of sensitivity accompanying the use of high- and even ultra-high resolution collimators should become more easily acceptable. Our experience provides support to this recommendation and we routinely employ the high-resolution parallel-hole collimators for all our $^{99m}$Tc studies with the GE/CGR Neurocam unless the patient is restless. Excellent anatomical representation of brain structures has been achieved with improved spatial resolution and hence reduced partial volume artefacts.

Fan beam collimators can further improve both resolution and sensitivity (Tsui et al. 1986). The geometric response functions for both fan beam and cone collimators have been derived based on an effective response function, which is determined by the geometric response of a single hole (Tsui and Gullberg 1990). The theoretical formulation provides a tool for the optimum design of fan beam collimators for SPET. The apparent system planar resolution improves by the magnification effect. Although the resolution deteriorates with increasing source to collimator distance for both parallel and fan beam collimators, it deteriorates less for fan beam. For a point source in air, the sensitivity of a parallel-hole collimator is depth-independent but that of fan beam increases as the source moves away from the collimator face.

A fundamental assumption in imaging is that the distribution of the radiopharmaceutical is stable during the data collection time; if it is not, artefacts are known to arise. This condition has traditionally guided the radiopharmaceutical chemists to develop compounds that exhibit suitably long equilibrium times. However, with the increased sensitivity of the three-headed systems, data collection times can become shorter and dynamic SPET studies can now be meaningfully performed. Radiopharmaceuticals that have a time-varying distribution reflecting a physiological process can now be developed for use with the new SPET machines.

With the increase in sensitivity offered by the new multiheaded imaging systems, the issues of patient throughput, reduced radiation exposure or improved accuracy can be addressed separately. It is now possible to decrease either the administered activity or data acquisition time, or to reach a compromise which, coupled with using high-resolution collimators, can yield improved image quality. The use of high-resolution collimators will result in an improvement in the reconstructed spatial resolution. The use of general-purpose collimators, coupled with the ease of patient positioning, will result in a greater patient throughput than currently achievable with a single rotating gamma camera. With such high-sensitivity systems, we anticipate that the role of SPET in routine and research studies will be enhanced.

The dose administered to the patient should be the lowest required to provide an adequate quality study in accordance with the radiation protection principle of 'as low as reasonably achievable' ALARA (ICRP 1988; DoH 1988). The newly developed multiheaded imaging systems primarily offer a significant increase in sensitivity. The optimum use of such a system can lead to improved image quality, increased patient throughput and dose reduction to the patient, staff and the general public. Thus, a more efficient utilization of administered radiopharmaceuticals to patients may be achieved.

# References

AAPM report no.22 (1987) Rotating scintillation camera SPECT acceptance testing and quality control. American Association of Physicists in Medicine, New York
Bailey DL, Hutton BF, Walker PJ (1987) Improved SPECT using simultaneous emission and transmission tomography. J Nucl Med 28:844–851
Budinger TF (1980) Physical attributes of single-photon tomography. J Nucl Med 21:579–592
Budinger TF (1990) Advances in emission tomography: Quo vadis? J Nucl Med 31:628–631
Chang LT (1978) A method for attenuation correction in radionuclide computed tomography. IEEE Trans Nucl Sci NS–25:638–643
DoH Publication (1988) Notes for guidance on the administration of radioactive substances to persons for the purposes of diagnosis, treatment or research. DoH, London
Fleming JS (1989) A technique for using CT images in attenuation correction and quantification in SPECT. Nucl Med Commun 10:83–97
Genna S, Smith AP (1988) The development of ASPECT, an annular single crystal brain camera for high efficiency SPECT. IEEE Trans Nucl Sci NS–35:654–658
Gilland DR, Tsui BMW, McCartney WH, et al (1990) Determination of the optimum filter function for SPECT imaging. J Nucl Med 29:643–650
Heller SL, Goodwin PN (1987) SPECT instrumentation: performance, lesion detection, and recent innovations. Semin Nucl Med 17:184–99
Herman GT (1980) Image reconstruction from projections: the fundamentals of computerized tomography. Academic Press, London
Higashi Y, Yamaoga N, Ohi J, et al (1985) Development of the Shimadzu single photon emission tomograph for head, SET–031. Shimadzu Rev 42:59–66
Holman BL, Carvalho PA, Zimmerman RE, et al (1990) Brain perfusion SPECT using an annular single crystal camera: initial clinical experience. J Nucl Med 31:1456–1561
Hor G (1988) Myocardial scintigraphy – 25 years after start. Eur J Nucl Med 13:619–636
Ichihara T (1990) Development of a high resolution SPECT system. Toshiba Med Rev 33:29–35
Ichihara T, Fujiki Y, Iwasaki T, et al (1990) High-spatial-resolution SPECT with fan beam collimators for brain imaging (Abstract). J Nucl Med 31:869
ICRP Publication 53 (1988) Radiation dose to patients from radiopharmaceuticals. Annals of the ICRP. Pergamon Press, Oxford
Jaszczak RJ, Chang LT, Murphy PH (1979) Single photon emission computed tomography using multi-slice fan beam collimators. IEEE Trans Nucl Sci 26:610–618
Jaszczak RJ, Greer KL, Floyd CE, et al (1984) Improved SPECT quantification using compensation of scattered photons. J Nucl Med 25:893–900
Jaszczak RJ, Floyd CE, Coleman RE (1985) Scatter compensation techniques for SPECT. IEEE Trans Nucl Sci NS–32:786–793
Keyes JW, Fahey FH, Harkness BA (1990) Tips for high quality SPECT. SNM Computer Instrumentation Council Newsletter, New York
Kimura K, Hashikawa K, Etani H, et al (1990) A new apparatus for brain imaging: a four-head rotating gamma camera single-photon emission computed tomograph. J Nucl Med 31:603–609
Koral KF, Swailem FM, Buchbinder S, et al (1990) SPECT dual-energy-window Compton correction: scatter multiplier required for quantification. J Nucl Med 31:90–98
Kouris K, Elgazzar A, Affana R, et al (1990) Methodology and performance assessment of zoom SPECT. J Nucl Med Technol 18:198–203
Kuhl DE, Edwards RQ (1963) Image separation in radioisotope scanning. Radiology 80:653–661
Kuhl DE, Alavi A, Reivich M, et al (1975) Computerized emission transaxial tomography and determination of local brain function. In: DeBlanc HJ, Sorenson JA (eds) Noninvasive brain imaging. Society of Nuclear Medicine, New York, pp 67–79
Lassen SA (1980) Gamma camera emission tomography: development and properties of a multi-sectional emission tomography system. Acta Radiol 363[Suppl]:1–75
Lassen NA, Sveinsdottir E, Kanno I, et al (1978) A fast single photon emission tomograph for regional cerebral blood flow studies in man. J Comput Assist Tomogr 2:660–661

Lim CB, Gottschalk S, Walker R, et al (1985) Triangular SPECT system for 3-D total organ volume imaging: design concept and preliminary results. IEEE Trans Nucl Sci 32:741–747

Lim CB, Walker R, Pinkstaff C, et al (1986) Triangular SPECT system for 3-D total organ volume imaging: performance results and dynamic imaging capability. IEEE Trans Nucl Sci 33:501–504

Malko JA, Van Heertum RL, Gullberg GT, et al (1986) SPECT liver imaging using an iterative attenuation correction algorithm and an external flood source. J Nucl Med 27:701–705

Matsuda H, Hisada K, Yamada M, et al (1990) Clinical applications of brain SPECT using the GCA–9300A. Toshiba Med Rev 33:36–42

Moore SC, Mueller SP (1986) Inversion of the 3-D Radon transform for a multidetector, point-focused SPECT brain scanner. Phys Med Biol 31:207–221

Mueller SP, Polak JF, Kijewski MF, et al (1986) Collimator selection for SPECT brain imaging: the advantage of high resolution. J Nucl Med 27:1729–1738

NEMA NU 1 (1986) Performance measurements of scintillation cameras. National Electrical Manufacturers Association

Radon J (1917) On the determination of functions from their integrals along certain manifolds. Math Phys Klasse 69:262–277

Sorenson JA, Phelps ME (1987) Physics in nuclear medicine, 2nd edn. Grune and Stratton, London

Stoddart HF, Stoddart HA (1979) A new development in single gamma transaxial tomography Union Carbide focused collimator scanner. IEEE Trans Nucl Sci 26:2710–2712

Tsui BMW, Gullberg GT (1990) The geometric transfer function for cone and fan beam collimators. Phys Med Biol 35:81–93

Tsui BMW, Gullberg GT, Edgerton ER, et al (1986) Design and clinical utility of a fan beam collimator for SPECT imaging of the head. J Nucl Med 27:810–819

Williams ED (ed) (1985) An introduction to emission computed tomography. Report no. 44. The Institute of Physical Sciences in Medicine, London

Chapter 4

# Clinical Use of SPET Imaging in Psychiatric and Neurological Disease

## Introduction

Recent advances in SPET technology have produced increased sensitivity and resolution of SPET systems (see Chaps. 2 and 3), allowing the technique to be applied in new and exciting ways to the understanding of clinical disease, particularly in the expanding fields of neurology and psychiatry. Functional neuroimaging has allowed clinicians to 'bypass the skull' and examine the active human brain in health and disease. SPET can aid doctors as never before as they make complex clinical decisions about patients.

In this chapter we provide an overview of how SPET can be of benefit in the clinical setting. For different diagnostic settings (e.g. dementias, cerebrovascular disease) we outline important points from various patients' histories, and include an explanation of their SPET findings. After each section we then provide a brief review of the published SPET work in this clinical area. Because this is a new field much of the active research, especially that pertaining to clinical syndromes, has not yet been published. We therefore often supplement the review of published material with our own clinical brain SPET experience.

## Normal Neuroanatomy and Neuroimaging

Below we demonstrate how SPET imaging of regional cerebral blood flow (rCBF) represents the normal human neuroanatomy. Transaxial sections of the normal human brain are shown (Fig. 1a), starting from the region of the brainstem and progressing upwards. For each level there is an MRI scan (on the left) representing the structural anatomy, and a $^{99m}$Tc-HMPAO (technetium-99m-D,L-hexamethylpropylene amine oxime) SPET scan (on the right) of a normal volunteer at the same level. Fig. 1b is a diagram representing the cerebral blood flow at that level, Neuroanatomical regions are labelled, and full explanations given in the legend. The transaxial images are followed by midsagittal and coronal images (Figs. 2 and 3).

## 52 NEUROACTIVATION AND NEUROIMAGING WITH SPET

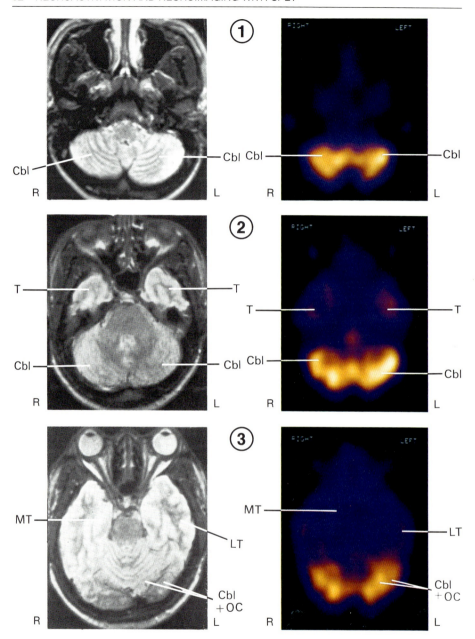

**Fig 1a.** Serial transaxial MRI scans on the left with corresponding HMPAO rCBF SPET maps on the right. From cerebellum (1) to cerebral cortex (8). Recognizable regions are labelled appropriately, as follows:

FC: Frontal Cortex  PC: Parietal Cortex  MPC: Motor Parietal Cortex  LT: Lateral Cortex  MT: Mesial Cortex Temporal Lobe  TH: Thalamus  CN: Caudate Nucleus  T: Temporal Lobe  PT: Posterior Temporal Lobe  BG: Basal Ganglia  CC: Corpus Callosum  VC: Visual Cortex  V: Lateral Ventricles  IC: Internal Capsule  OC: Occipital Cortex  WM: White Matter  Cbl: Cerebellum

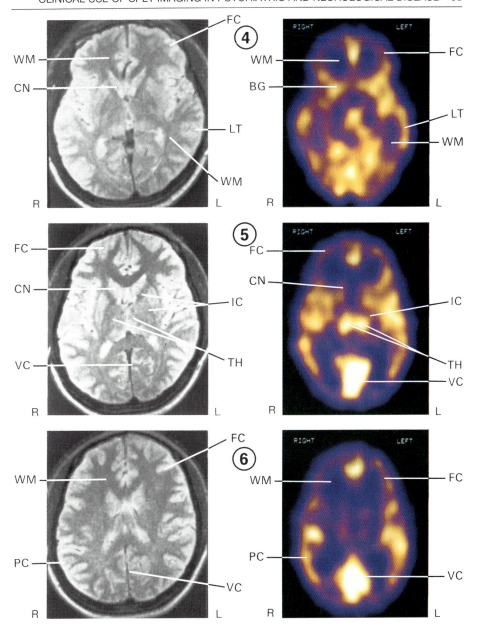

**Fig 1a (contd).** Serial transaxial MRI scans on the left with corresponding HMPAO rCBF SPET maps on the right. From cerebellum (1) to cerebral cortex (8). Recognizable regions are labelled appropriately, as follows:

FC: Frontal Cortex   PC: Parietal Cortex   MPC: Motor Parietal Cortex   LT: Lateral Cortex   MT: Mesial Cortex Temporal Lobe   TH: Thalamus   CN: Caudate Nucleus   T: Temporal Lobe   PT: Posterior Temporal Lobe   BG: Basal Ganglia   CC: Corpus Callosum   VC: Visual Cortex   V: Lateral Ventricles   IC: Internal Capsule   OC: Occipital Cortex   WM: White Matter   Cbl: Cerebellum

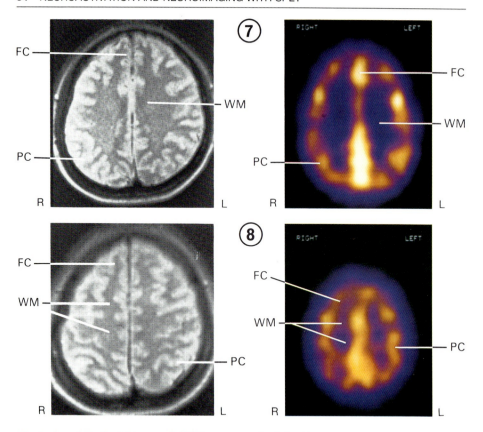

**Fig 1a (contd).** Serial transaxial MRI scans on the left with corresponding HMPAO rCBF SPET maps on the right. From cerebellum (1) to cerebral cortex (8). Recognizable regions are labelled appropriately, as follows:

FC: Frontal Cortex  PC: Parietal Cortex  MPC: Motor Parietal Cortex  LT: Lateral Cortex  MT: Mesial Cortex Temporal Lobe  TH: Thalamus  CN: Caudate Nucleus  T: Temporal Lobe  PT: Posterior Temporal Lobe  BG: Basal Ganglia  CC: Corpus Callosum  VC: Visual Cortex  V: Lateral Ventricles  IC: Internal Capsule  OC: Occipital Cortex  WM: White Matter  Cbl: Cerebellum

**Fig 1b.** Drawings of X-ray computed tomography cuts with Brodmann's areas marked ▶ on left and vascular territories on right. Blue indicates branches of anterior cerebral artery; red, middle cerebral artery; yellow, posterior cerebral artery; and green, internal carotid artery. AI indicates anterior internal frontal; MI, middle internal frontal; PI, posterior internal frontal; PAC, paracentral; IP, superior and interior internal parietal; HA, Heubner's artery; CC, arteries of corpus callosum (small branches of either pericallosal artery or medial branch of posterior cerebral artery); PF, prefrontal; PC, precentral; CS, central sulcus; PP, anterior and posterior parietal; AN, angular; AT, anterior temporal; MT, middle temporal; PT, posterior temporal; TO, temporo-occipital; LS, lenticulostriate; IB, insular branches (small branches of major branches of middle cerebral artery); LB, lateral branch (includes temporal branches); MB, medial branch (includes calcarine and parieto-occipital arteries); THP, thalamoperforation, thalamogeniculate, and posterior choroidal; and ACH, anterior choroidal and additional small branches of internal carotid artery. (Courtesy of Dr Hanna Damasio; Arch. Neurol. 1983;40:138–142)

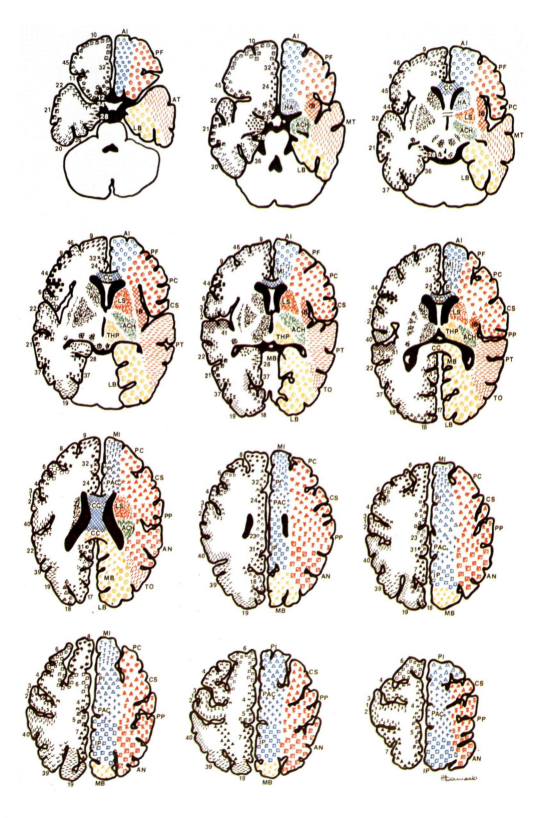

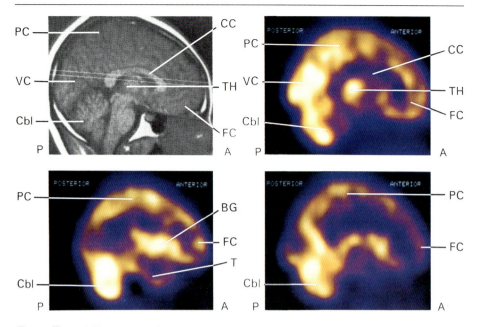

**Fig 2.** The midline sagittal MRI scan (top left) and corresponding HMPAO rCBF SPET image (top right) and representative left and right hemisphere sagittal sections of the flow study are shown. Recognizable regions are labelled appropriately, as follows:

FC: Frontal Cortex  PC: Parietal Cortex  MPC: Motor Parietal Cortex  LT: Lateral Cortex  MT: Mesial Cortex Temporal Lobe  TH: Thalamus  CN: Caudate Nucleus  T: Temporal Lobe  PT: Posterior Temporal Lobe  BG: Basal Ganglia  CC: Corpus Callosum  VC: Visual Cortex  V: Lateral Ventricles  IC: Internal Capsule  OC: Occipital Cortex  WM: White Matter  Cbl: Cerebellum

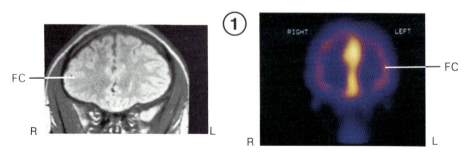

**Fig 3. (above to facing page)** Coronal MRI scans (left) and corresponding HMPAO rCBF SPET maps (right) progressing from frontal (1) to posterior (5). Recognizable regions are labelled appropriately, as follows:

FC: Frontal Cortex  PC: Parietal Cortex  MPC: Motor Parietal Cortex  LT: Lateral Cortex  MT: Mesial Cortex Temporal Lobe  TH: Thalamus  CN: Caudate Nucleus  T: Temporal Lobe  PT: Posterior Temporal Lobe  BG: Basal Ganglia  CC: Corpus Callosum  VC: Visual Cortex  V: Lateral Ventricles  IC: Internal Capsule  OC: Occipital Cortex  WM: White Matter  Cbl: Cerebellum

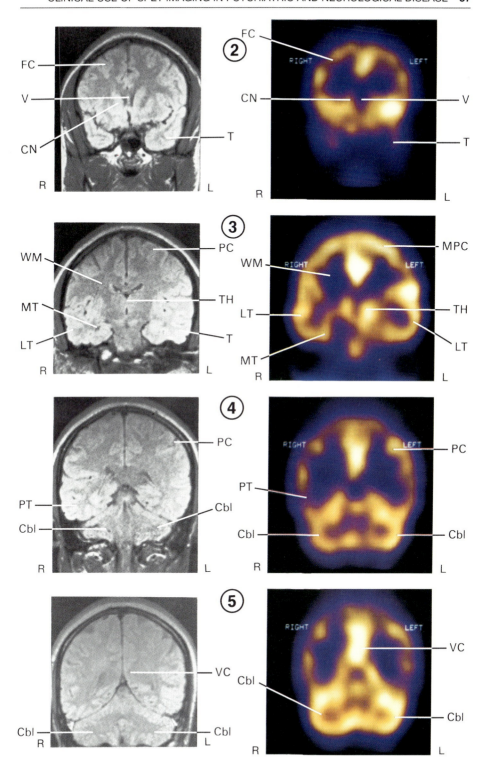

**Fig 4.** Midline sagittal MRI scan (top left) with corresponding rCBF SPET image (top right). Note the severely decreased frontal cortical perfusion. Transverse SPET images (bottom right and left) reveal the characteristic AD pattern of decreased perfusion to frontal, posterior temporal and parietal regions.

# Dementia

Dementia affects 5% of those over age 65 and 25% of those more than 80 years old (Terry and Katzman 1983). As the demographic make-up of Western countries ages, the diagnosis and treatment of demented patients will represent an ever-expanding component of total health care expense.

SPET neuroimaging will play an important role in tackling this massive public health problem (Holman and Tumeh 1990). High-resolution SPET is one of the most effective clinical tests for distinguishing between different dementia syndromes. Unfortunately, there are currently only a few clearly treatable and reversible causes of dementia. Thus, at present, the most important reasons for making a proper diagnosis of the aetiology of dementia are for prognosis, family counselling, and to exclude the treatable causes (e.g. tertiary syphilis, normal-pressure hydrocephalus, vitamin $B_{12}$ deficiency, depression). However, new therapies for dementia are being actively investigated. Once these become available, making an effective diagnosis with SPET neuroimaging will become of even greater importance.

## Alzheimer's Disease

### CASE 1

*Clinical Case History*

This 86-year-old man had been in good health and with intact intellectual functions when it was noticed that he had a change in his personality and decreased memory and other cognitive skills. The decline started approximately 2 years before his scan. His neurological examination was normal and he had no family history of dementing illnesses. A SPET scan was done to help with his diagnosis.

DIAGNOSIS: Alzheimer's disease

*Image Acquisition Parameters*

The patient was given intravenous 718 MBq $^{99m}$Tc-HMPAO. He was scanned supine on the GE/CGR Neurocam for 15 minutes (128 projections in a 64 × 64 matrix acquisition) using high-resolution collimators. Tomographic slices were reconstructed in the transaxial, coronal and sagittal planes using a Hanning prefilter with 1.0 cycles/cm cut-off frequency, a Ramp filter and attenuation correction (Fig. 4).

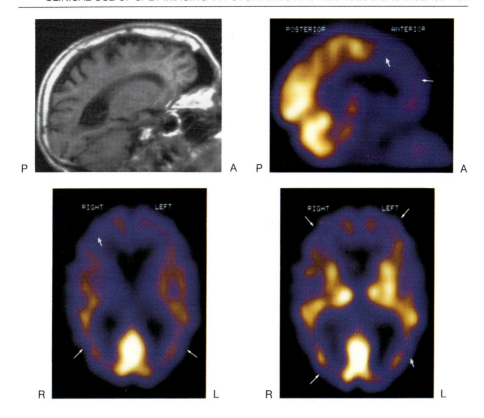

## CASE 2

*Clinical Case History*

This 74-year-old male was sent for SPET scanning because of a history of a gradual decline in memory and other cognitive functions over 10 months. He was normotensive with no focal signs on neurological examination. There was no pertinent family history.

DIAGNOSIS: Alzheimer's disease

*Image Acquisition Parameters*

The patient was given intravenous 690 MBq $^{99m}$Tc-HMPAO. He was scanned supine on the GE/CGR Neurocam for 15 minutes (128 projections in a 64 × 64 matrix acquisition) using high-resolution collimators. Tomographic slices were reconstructed in the transaxial, coronal and sagittal planes using a Hanning prefilter with 1.0 cycles/cm cut-off frequency, a Ramp filter and attenuation correction (Fig. 5).

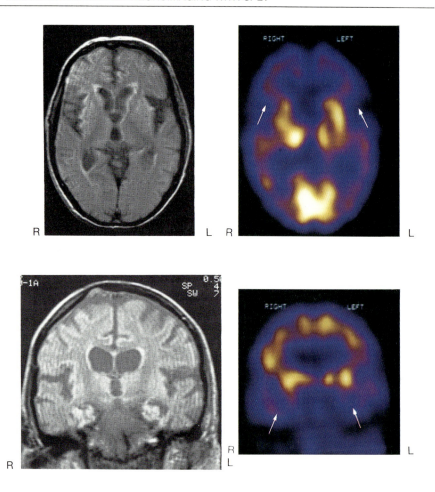

**Fig 5.** Transverse sections at the level of the basal ganglia (MRI, top left; SPET, top right). The SPET image demonstrates reduced perfusion to the frontal, temporal and posterior parietal lobes. Coronal sections through the mid-temporal lobe (MRI bottom left; SPET bottom right). The SPET image reveals decreased bi-temporal perfusion sometimes seen in AD.

## CASE 3

### Clinical Case History

This 79-year-old woman suffered a gradual decline in her memory and other cognitive functions over 3 years. She had no family history of dementia and was otherwise in good health. Her physical examination was normal except for her poor cognitive skills.

DIAGNOSIS: Alzheimer's disease

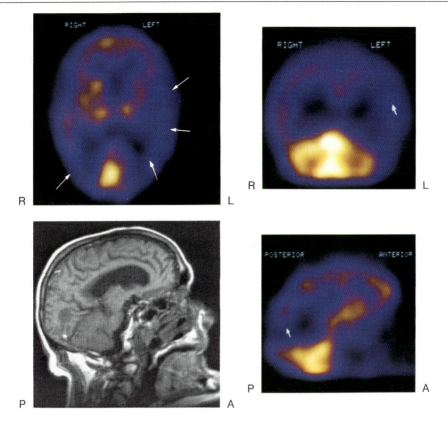

**Fig 6.** Clockwise (from top left), selected transaxial, posterior coronal, and right paramedial sagittal SPET flow maps and a midline sagittal MRI tomogram are shown. There is marked reduction of perfusion to the parietal and temporal lobes which, although bilateral, is worse on the left.

## Image Acquisition Parameters

The patient was given intravenous 777 MBq $^{99m}$Tc-HMPAO. She was scanned supine on the GE/CGR Neurocam for 15 minutes (128 projections in a 64 × 64 matrix acquisition) using high-resolution collimators. Tomographic slices were reconstructed in the transaxial, coronal and sagittal planes using a Hanning prefilter with 1.0 cycles/cm cut-off frequency, a Ramp filter and attenuation correction (Fig. 6).

## Comment

The most frequently reported SPET findings in Alzheimer's disease (AD) are bilateral hypoperfusion and hypometabolism of the parietal and temporal lobes (Holman 1986; Gemmell et al. 1987; Burns et al. 1989; Montaldi et al. 1990; Neary et al 1990; Johnson et al. 1991). The sensorimotor and occipital regions are usually spared and appear normal. As the disease progresses, the frontal lobes sometimes become involved as well, showing decreased perfusion and metabolism. Although most cases of AD show bilateral involvement, in a small percentage of patients the findings are unilateral (Terry and Katzman 1983).

This uniform finding of decreased temporal and parietal rCBF perfusion in AD makes SPET a useful tool for evaluating a patient with dementia (Johnson et al. 1991). AD has a distinct neuroSPET picture. The other common dementias – multi-infarct dementia, Binswanger's disease, AIDS, and pseudo-dementia of depression – are usually readily distinguishable from AD with SPET neuroimaging. This is important for prognosis, and may become more important once an effective therapy for AD is found.

How sensitive (ability to detect all patients with AD) and specific (ability to not include people who do not have AD) is high-resolution SPET for AD? Johnson et al. (1991) studied 58 AD patients and 15 age-matched healthy controls using SPET with iodoamphetamine ($^{123}$I-IMP). Assessed qualitatively, SPET scans were found to be 88% sensitive and 87% specific for diagnosing AD. Using region-of-interest semi-quantitative analysis the parietal lobes were found to be the most severely affected in AD, and parietal lobe hypometabolism was correlated with dementia rating scales.

In another AD study, using $^{99m}$Tc-HMPAO, Burns et al. (1989) also found a connection between poor performance on specific neuropsychological tests and decreased rCBF in pertinent brain areas. Studying 20 AD subjects and 6 age-matched healthy controls, they found that AD patients had lower rCBF in the temporal and posterior parietal lobes compared with controls. Additionally, within the AD groups correlations were found between neuropsychological tests and rCBF: praxis correlated with poor posterior parietal activity, deficient memory with decreased left temporal activity, and declining language skills with decreased activity throughout the left hemisphere. SPET, although able to detect subtle changes in AD, has some limitations. Reed et al. (1989) performed SPET scans in 21 mildly demented AD subjects. In 5 of these SPET images of the parietal and temporal lobes were normal even though these same subjects performed poorly on memory tests. They concluded that clinical AD and cortical neuropathology may precede the characteristic SPET picture.

In summary, SPET imaging is a useful adjunct in establishing the diagnosis of AD. Additionally, the neuroSPET image often correlates with the specific cognitive deficits displayed by the patient. In the future, as effective therapies for AD emerge, neuroSPET imaging will almost certainly play a role in predicting and evaluating response to treatment. Chap. 10 reviews how SPET imaging of pharmacological activation of AD patients may help evaluate response to treatment.

## Teaching Point

> Clinically, Alzheimer's disease often presents with a history of a gradual decline in cognitive functions. Dramatic, sharp changes in intellect are more likely to represent a vascular or infectious process than AD. The typical SPET pattern in AD demonstrates a reduction of perfusion to the temporal and parietal lobes bilaterally. Two important points to remember are that: (1) in later stages of the disease the frontal lobes can also be involved; and (2) some cases of AD have asymmetric involvement.

## Multi-Infarct Dementia

### CASE 1

*Clinical Case History*

This 65-year-old woman suffered cognitive deterioration following a left brain stroke 7 years previously. Six months before her scan she suffered a right brain stroke with further intellectual decline. She had angina and hypertension. Physical examination revealed mild weakness of her left hand and arm.

DIAGNOSIS: Multi-infarct dementia

*Image Acquisition Parameters*

The patient was given intravenous 700 MBq $^{99m}$Tc-HMPAO. She was scanned supine on the GE/CGR Neurocam for 15 minutes (128 projections in a 64 × 64 matrix acquisition) using high-resolution collimators. Tomographic slices were reconstructed in the transaxial, coronal and sagittal planes using a Hanning prefilter with 1.0 cycles/cm cut-off frequency, a Ramp filter and attenuation correction (Fig. 7).

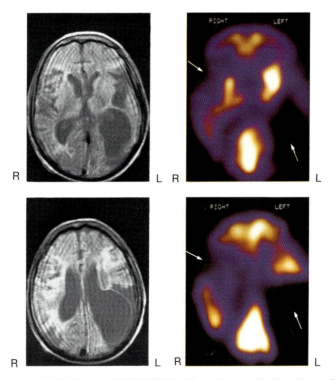

**Fig 7.** Transverse MRI (left) and rCBF SPET (right) sections at the basal ganglia (top) and mid-ventricular (bottom) levels. Multiple foci of marked perfusion deficits in both hemispheres are readily apparent.

## CASE 2

*Clinical Case History*

This 82-year-old woman suffered a gradual step-wise reduction in her intellectual functions over 3 years in association with intermittent transient ischaemic attacks (TIAs). She had hypertension and her neurological examination was non-focal.

DIAGNOSIS: Multi-infarct dementia

*Image Acquisition Parameters*

The patient was given intravenous 760 MBq $^{99m}$Tc-HMPAO. She was scanned supine on the GE/CGR Neurocam for 15 minutes (128 projections in a 64 × 64 matrix acquisition) using high-resolution collimators. Tomographic slices were reconstructed in the transaxial, coronal and sagittal planes using a Hanning prefilter with 1.0 cycles/cm cut-off frequency, a Ramp filter and attenuation correction (Fig. 8).

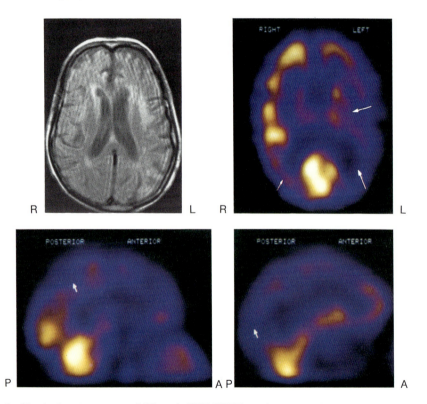

**Fig 8.** Clockwise, transverse MRI and rCBF SPET sections rostral to the basal ganglia (top), and two rCBF sagittal SPET sections (right and left paramedian midline). These demonstrate multiple perfusion deficits best seen in the left parietal lobe and both posterior temporal lobes. The pattern is compatible with MID.

## CASE 3

*Clinical Case History*

This 80-year-old man had a loss of intellectual function, occurring at discrete intervals over several years. His neurological examination was non-focal. He had hypertension and a family history of heart disease.

DIAGNOSIS: Multi-infarct dementia

*Image Acquisition Parameters*

The patient was given intravenous 724 MBq $^{99m}$Tc-HMPAO. He was scanned supine on the GE/CGR Neurocam for 15 minutes (128 projections in a 64 × 64 matrix acquisition) using high-resolution collimators. Tomographic slices were reconstructed in the transaxial, coronal and sagittal planes using a Hanning prefilter with 1.0 cycles/cm cut-off frequency, a Ramp filter and attenuation correction (Fig. 9).

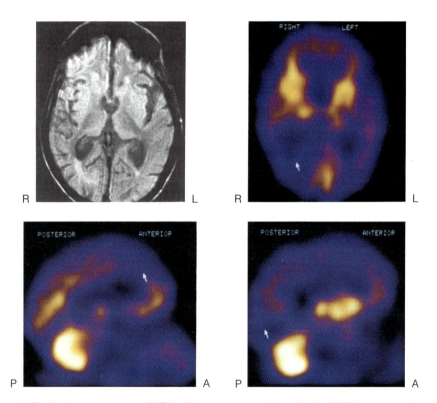

**Fig 9.** Clockwise, transverse MRI with a corresponding rCBF SPET study, and two separate sagittal flow maps (right paramedian, left paramedian) shown to highlight areas of impaired perfusion (arrows) typical of MID. The right posterior temporal infarction is seen both on MRI and SPET. Note that the sagittal SPET sections demonstrate well the other perfusion deficits.

*Comment*

Several studies have now established the efficacy of SPET in making the diagnosis of multi-infarct dementia (MID) (Ell et al. 1985; Gemmell et al. 1987; Cohen et al. 1989). The distinctive SPET pattern of MID – patchy areas of hypoperfusion corresponding to infarcted tissue – makes SPET a sensitive tool for diagnosis. In later chapters we will see how SPET may be used to evaluate vasodilators and other treatments used in MID.

*Teaching Point*

> The SPET image in MID is one of patchy distribution of the tracer with numerous perfusion deficits corresponding to impaired tracer uptake in infarcted tissue. This is usually accompanied by a clinical history of a step-wise reduction in intellectual functions. Often MID patients also have multiple risk factors for cerebrovascular disease (e.g. family history, hypertension, elevated cholesterol levels).

## Frontal Dementias

### CASE 1

*Clinical Case History*

This 65-year-old woman had had a frontal lobotomy 30 years previously for the treatment of psychosis. She now had a progressive memory loss and choreiform movements.

DIAGNOSIS: Probable frontal dementia secondary to lobotomy

*Image Acquisition Parameters*

The patient was given intravenous 710 MBq $^{99m}$Tc-HMPAO. She was scanned supine on the GE/CGR Neurocam for 15 minutes (128 projections in a 64 × 64 matrix acquisition) using high-resolution collimators. Tomographic slices were reconstructed in the transaxial, coronal and sagittal planes using a Hanning prefilter with 1.0 cycles/cm cut-off frequency, a Ramp filter and attenuation correction (Fig. 10).

*Comment*

Several rare dementias constitute the category of frontal dementias. The most well-recognized of these is Pick's disease, characterized by a speech disturbance, personality change and progressive dementia. SPET scans in these conditions show hypoperfusion in the frontal lobes, with relatively intact perfusion in the rest of the cortex. The case described above, although not an example of this group of diseases, displays iatrogenic frontal lobe syndrome, produced by the surgical operation which severed the fibres projecting to the frontal lobe running through the orbitofrontal cortex.

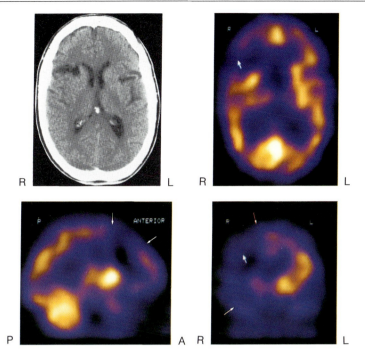

**Fig 10.** Clockwise, a transverse CT study is shown with a corresponding transaxial flow map, coronal and right paramedian sagittal flow templates. The limited surgical defect displayed on the CT study leads to a more significant flow abnormality, which is extensive. The abnormal right frontal lobe, although present, is disconnected and dysfunctional.

Frontal lobe dementias are also seen in other conditions. For example, Neary et al. (1990) found a frontal lobe dementia in many patients suffering from amyotrophic lateral sclerosis – a disease which was previously thought to be confined to the anterior horn cells of the spinal cord. SPET neuroimaging can help in verifying the diagnosis of frontal lobe dementias.

## Teaching Point

SPET scans show hypoperfusion of the frontal lobes in patients with frontal dementias. The SPET scan picture of the frontal dementias is similar to that seen in depressed patients. The two conditions must then be distinguished on clinical and other grounds. Patients with Pick's disease often have a characteristic speech pattern that can be helpful in making this distinction.

The case above illustrates the important point that rCBF perfusion deficits may be caused by two different types of neuropathology: (1) loss of underlying tissue as in atrophy or infarction, or (2) brain tissue being present but non-functioning. A functional change visible on rCBF SPET imaging may thus stem from a structural problem (infarction or atrophy) or may reflect present but malfunctioning brain regions, as in epilepsy or this case of a frontal dementia. rCBF perfusion deficits and atrophy are independent but may coexist.

## Acquired Immune Deficiency Syndrome (AIDS) Dementia

### CASE 1

*Clinical Case History*

This 37-year-old man with known human immunodeficiency virus (HIV) infection suddenly had a tonic-clonic seizure. He had no previous history of head trauma or seizures. His physical examination after recovery from the seizures was non-focal. Results of general metabolic tests, lumbar puncture and cranial CT were normal. Friends noted that he had suffered a change in personality over the previous 4 months. He himself noted subjective memory impairment over the previous 3 months.

DIAGNOSIS: AIDS dementia

*Image Acquisition Parameters*

The patient was given intravenous 760 MBq $^{99m}$Tc-HMPAO. He was scanned supine on the GE/CGR Neurocam for 15 minutes (128 projections in a 64 × 64 matrix acquisition) using high-resolution collimators. Tomographic slices were reconstructed in the transaxial, coronal and sagittal planes using a Hanning prefilter with 1.0 cycles/cm cut-off frequency, a Ramp filter and attenuation correction (Fig. 11).

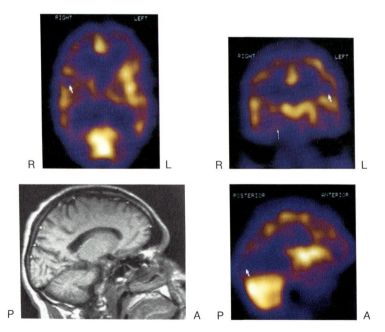

**Fig 11.** Clockwise, flow maps in transverse, coronal and left sagittal planes, with a mid-sagittal MRI study are shown. Whilst the MRI study shows atrophy, the rCBF SPET study shows multiple discrete but small areas of impaired perfusion.

## CASE 2

### Clinical Case History

This 41-year-old man with known HIV infection had an episode lasting 1 hour of sudden dysphasia, confusion and clumsiness. He recovered fully. Neurological examination revealed brisk reflexes on the right side.

DIAGNOSIS: AIDS dementia

### Image Acquisition Parameters

The patient was given intravenous 760 MBq $^{99m}$Tc-HMPAO. He was scanned supine on the GE/CGR Neurocam for 15 minutes (128 projections in a 64 × 64 matrix acquisition) using high-resolution collimators. Tomographic slices were reconstructed in the transaxial, coronal and sagittal planes using a Hanning prefilter with 1.0 cycles/cm cut-off frequency, a Ramp filter and attenuation correction (Fig. 12).

### Comment

The SPET abnormalities seen in patients with HIV and HIV-dementia are essentially non-specific. Patients with a space-occupying lesion caused by an infection or malignancy will probably display a perfusion deficit on rCBF SPET

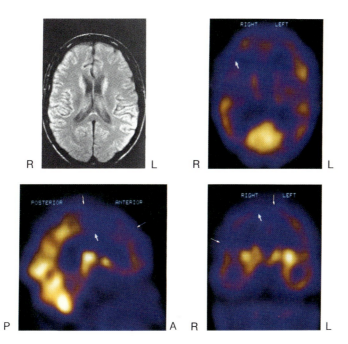

**Fig 12.** Clockwise, a transaxial MRI and corresponding flow map, and a coronal and midline sagittal HMPAO flow map are shown. Whilst the MRI study is normal there are major perfusion deficits (see arrows).

scanning. Other HIV patients show diffusely decreased perfusion in the parieto-temporal region (Costa et al. 1988). Yet other HIV-dementia patients display patchy hypoperfusion similar to a multi-infarct pattern. Importantly, SPET scanning can be markedly abnormal even in the face of normal structural neuroimaging, thus demonstrating diffuse neuronal damage by HIV.

*Teaching Point*

> SPET scans of patients with HIV dementia can sometimes be abnormal even when MRI or CT neuroimaging is normal. In some patients the pattern of patchy perfusion deficits may resemble the rCBF SPET scan pattern of a patient with multi-infarct dementia.

## Normal Pressure Hydrocephalus

### CASE 1

*Clinical Case History*

This 55-year-old woman was in good health until 2 years previously when she began having difficulty walking. She noted that she walked slowly and had difficulty turning. One year after this friends and family noted that her memory was worse and that she was more irritable than before. Physical examination revealed increased motor tone in her legs bilaterally, worse on her right. She had been incontinent of urine for the past 3 months.

DIAGNOSIS: Normal pressure hydrocephalus

*Image Acquisition Parameters*

The patient was given intravenous 680 MBq $^{99m}$Tc-HMPAO. She was scanned supine on the GE/CGR Neurocam for 15 minutes (128 projections in a 64 × 64 matrix acquisition) using high-resolution collimators. Tomographic slices were reconstructed in the transaxial, coronal and sagittal planes using a Hanning prefilter with 1.0 cycles/cm cut-off frequency, a Ramp filter and attenuation correction (Fig. 13).

*Comment*

Normal pressure hydrocephalus is one of the treatable dementias, recognized by the characteristic triad of a gait disorder, intellectual decline and incontinence. In some patients, shunting of CSF can help restore gait, continence and occasionally intellectual function. rCBF SPET experience with this condition is limited at present. Interestingly, normal pressure hydrocephalus was one of the first dementias in which nuclear medicine was used as an aid in diagnosis. Injection of radioactive tracers into the CSF with serial scans over several days can give an estimate of CSF diffusion and uptake, which are impaired in this disease.

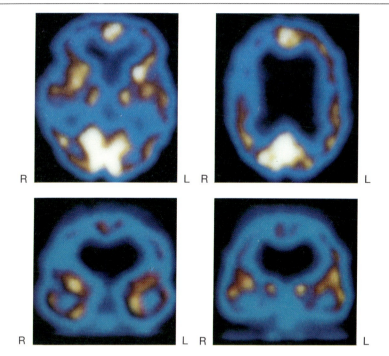

**Fig 13.** Clockwise, two transverse and two coronal blood flow maps are shown. These demonstrate decreased perfusion globally, with an appearance suggestive of enlarged ventricles.

## Teaching Point

Structural abnormalities in normal pressure hydrocephalus can sometimes be recognized on rCBF SPET scanning, as in this case. When a diffuse rCBF abnormality is noted on SPET scanning, CT or MRI should be performed to examine structural pathology.

## Cortical–Basal Degeneration

### CASE 1

*Clinical Case History*

A 76-year-old woman presented with a 2-year history of progressive apraxia of her right hand. More recently similar signs had developed in the left hand. In addition there was mild bradykinesia and rigidity in both arms, more pronounced on the right. She was intellectually intact. She was thought clinically to display evidence of focal cortical and focal basal ganglia degeneration.

DIAGNOSIS: Focal cortical–basal degeneration

## Image Acquisition Parameters

The patient was given intravenous 600 MBq $^{99m}$Tc-HMPAO. She was scanned supine on the GE/CGR Neurocam for 15 minutes (128 projections in a 64 × 64 matrix acquisition) using high-resolution collimators. Tomographic slices were reconstructed in the transaxial, coronal and sagittal planes using a Hanning prefilter with 1.0 cycles/cm cut-off frequency, a Ramp filter and attenuation correction (Fig. 14).

## Comment

Cortical–basal degenerative syndromes are rare disorders in which patients exhibit normal muscle power but have an inability to initiate their movements properly. They have a combination of extrapyramidal rigidity or tremor along with signs of corticospinal disease. These idiopathic diseases are usually relentless and patients eventually succumb to the medical complications of their inability to initiate movements. Some patients, although not all, develop dementia.

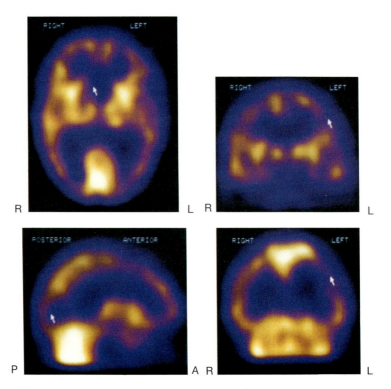

**Fig 14.** Clockwise, transverse, anterior coronal, posterior coronal and right sagittal flow maps are shown. The arrows point to cortical and basal ganglia perfusion abnormalities in this patient with a normal CT.

# Paediatric Development Disorders

SPET scanning shows promise in diagnosing and understanding developmental disorders occurring in early childhood and infancy. As a group, these disorders are poorly understood and categorized (Adams and Victor 1986).

Cerebral palsy has long been a frustrating disorder for physicians. It was often difficult to predict the long-term prognosis in a young child. In addition, results of structural imaging (CT and MRI) are often normal, despite the obvious pathology displayed by the patient. A puzzling clinical question has always been why cerebral palsy takes different forms (e.g. hemiplegia, diplegia, triplegia or tetraplegia). Denays et al. (1990) used $^{99m}$Tc-HMPAO SPET to study 13 subjects with cerebral palsy and found that these various subgroups had differing SPET images. Subjects with mild diplegia had normal SPET images. Those with hemiplegia had contralateral cortical hypoperfusion. SPET showed bilateral hypoperfusion in the superior motor cortex in subjects with moderate di- or tetraplegia. Subjects with *severe* di- or tetraplegia had bilateral hypoperfusion in the superior and inferior motor *and* prefrontal and parietal cortices.

SPET studies have also been used to help in the understanding of congenital dysphasias, dyslexias and attention-deficit and hyperactivity disorder (ADHD) (Denays et al. 1989; Lou et al. 1990). One of the more interesting ways in which SPET can be used to understand human development is to study a progression of images obtained as infants mature, corresponding to brain maturation and development. Rubinstein et al. (1989) retrospectively studied the $^{123}$I-IMP SPET images of 30 babies who had had a normal clinical examination, EEG and CT at the time of SPET imaging. Before age 2 months there was marked predominance of the thalamic perfusion relative to the rest of the cortex. The distribution and development of regional cortical activity followed a strict sequence. At age 40 weeks parietal and occipital lobe activity appeared. Frontal lobe activity first appeared at age 2 months and did not reach an adult pattern until 2 years.

SPET imaging thus holds promise for better understanding of human development, both in health and in disease.

# Infantile Autism

One of the most enigmatic childhood development disorders is infantile autism. This tragic behavioural disorder with its characteristic pattern of language and social arrest accompanied by stereotyped behaviour is poorly understood.

## CASE 1

### Clinical Case History

This 25-year-old man had a normal birth and delivery. He progressed normally in his motor development until approximately age 18 months when he stopped walking and became reclusive with little interaction with others. He never developed language beyond saying a simple 'yes' or 'no'. He had always been intolerant of change and had frequent stereotyped movements which he repeated throughout the day. Numerous clinical investigations (EEG, serology) had been carried out throughout his life, all of which had been negative. There was no pertinent family history. A cranial CT scan was normal.

DIAGNOSIS: Infantile autism

## Image Acquisition Parameters

The patient was given intravenous 10 MBq/kg $^{99m}$Tc-HMPAO. He was scanned supine on the GE/CGR Neurocam for 15 minutes (128 projections in a 64 × 64 matrix acquisition) using high-resolution collimators. Tomographic slices were reconstructed in the transaxial, coronal and sagittal planes using a Hanning prefilter with 1.0 cycles/cm cut-off frequency, a Ramp filter and attenuation correction (Fig. 15).

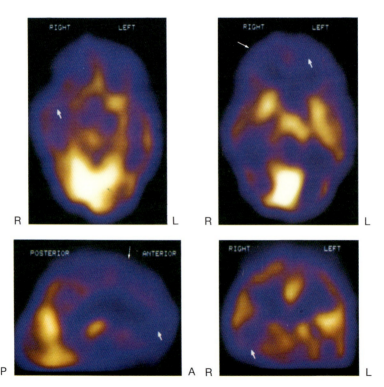

**Fig 15.** Clockwise, low and high transverse, coronal and left sagittal flow maps are shown. There is decreased perfusion to the left and right frontal and right temporal lobes.

## CASE 2

### Clinical Case History

This 28-year-old man had a normal gestation and birth. His mother noted at an early age that he was more irritable than her other children. At the age of 1 year she took the child to a physician for evaluation because of his failure to interact well with her. The patient never developed language skills above a rudimentary level. Numerous investigations (CT, EEG, serology) had all been normal. He had frequent repetitive movements, was intolerant of change, and did not engage in formal play or interact well with others.

DIAGNOSIS: Infantile autism

### Image Acquisition Parameters

The patient was given intravenous 10 MBq/kg $^{99m}$Tc-HMPAO. He was scanned supine on the GE/CGR Neurocam for 25 minutes (128 projections in a 64 × 64 matrix acquisition) using high-resolution collimators. Tomographic slices were reconstructed in the transaxial, coronal and sagittal planes using a Hanning prefilter with 0.8 cycles/cm cut-off frequency, a Ramp filter and attenuation correction (Fig. 16).

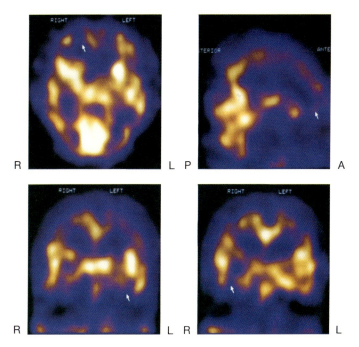

**Fig 16.** Clockwise, transverse, midline sagittal and two coronal flow maps are shown. These images are unusually noisy because of the need for rapid acquisition of data (5 minutes total) caused by poor patient cooperation. There is global depression in blood flow to the entire cortex (see text). The arrows point to representative areas of focally decreased perfusion.

## Comment

Recently, MRI scans of patients with infantile autism have revealed hypoplasia of cerebellar vermal lobules VI and VII (Courchesne et al. 1988; Murakami et al. 1989), and developmental abnormalities in the forebrain (Gaffney et al. 1989), brainstem (Hashimoto et al. 1989) and other parts of the cortex (Piven et al. 1990). Many believe that these abnormalities derive from abnormal neuronal development and migration (Plioplys et al. 1990).

One would expect PET and SPET to demonstrate how these structural and developmental abnormalities affect a functioning autistic brain. PET studies to date have had conflicting results, with some researchers finding a global increase in cortical metabolism in autistic patients using $^{18}$FDG (Rumsey et al. 1985; Horwitz et al. 1988), and others not (Herold et al. 1988). One PET study found impaired interactions between frontal/parietal regions and the neostriatum and thalamus in autistic patients (Horwitz et al. 1988).

Table 1. Summary of functional neuroimaging studies in autism

| Study | Method | n | IQ | Scanning environment | Conclusions |
|---|---|---|---|---|---|
| Rumsey et al. (1985) | $^{18}$FDG PET | 10 A[a]<br>15 C | 7: 80–120<br>3: <80 | Sensory-deprived, ears plugged, 150 minutes | A 20% > C for glucose metabolism |
| Horwitz et al. (1988) | $^{18}$FDG PET | 14 A[b]<br>14 C | 11: 80–126<br>3: <80 | Sensory-deprived | A 12% > C for glucose metabolism. Decreased frontal and parietal interactions in autism |
| Heh et al. (1989) | $^{18}$FDG PET | 7 A<br>8 C | Av. 90 | 100 minutes, dark room, continuous performance test | No differences |
| Herold et al. (1988) | $^{18}$FDG PET and $^{15}$O$_2$ PET | 6 A<br>6–8 C | 3: <80 | Dark room, relaxed, listening to favourite music | $^{18}$FDG: no difference. $^{15}$O$_2$: decreased rates in A, not statistically significant |
| Sherman et al. (1984) | Xenon-133 single photon | 7 A<br>13 C | 30–76 | Dark, quiet room | Decreased mean rCBF in A (C: 79 ml/100 g/min; A, 68 ml/100 g/min) |

[a] A = autistic; C = controls
[b] 10 of these subjects were the same as in Rumsey et al. (1985)

Only one published single photon (non-tomographic) study has been carried out in autistic patients, despite the availability of appropriate tracers. This study found diffuse decreases in cortical metabolism using xenon-133 (Sherman et al. 1984) (Table 1).

We recently performed a pilot study at the UCMSM on 8 subjects (4 patients with infantile autism and 4 controls) using high-resolution rCBF SPET with $^{99m}$Tc-HMPAO (George et al. 1991a). The autism group had lower perfusion in all brain regions after normalization for dose (Table 2). This decreased perfusion ranged from 58% to 72% of the corresponding perfusion rates in controls. The differences were all statistically significant ($p = 0.02$, Mann-Whitney test).

In addition to the global decrease in brain perfusion, the autism group had focally decreased perfusion in the right lateral temporal and right, left and mid-frontal lobes (Table 3). Ratios for basal ganglia and other temporal lobe regions did not significantly differ between the two groups.

The decreased right lateral temporal and frontal lobe perfusion in the autism group is readily apparent on qualitative analysis of the individual scans, and thus may have important diagnostic as well as research implications (Fig. 17). Moreover, right temporal and frontal hypometabolism correlates with the global behavioural disturbances of autism. The temporal lobes play an important role in language (Penfield and Rasmussen 1950), while the frontal lobes are important for higher planning and social interaction (Stuss and Benson 1986). As noted above, both behaviours are abnormal in autism.

Table 2. Significant region-of-interest perfusion ratios and $p$ values[a] in autistic subjects compared with controls

| Region of brain | Autism ($n = 4$) Mean | Controls ($n = 4$) Mean | $p$ value |
| --- | --- | --- | --- |
| Right frontal/ visual cortex | 0.68 | 0.79 | 0.020 |
| Left frontal/ visual cortex | 0.66 | 0.82 | 0.020 |
| Mid-frontal/ visual cortex | 0.83 | 0.99 | 0.020 |
| Right lateral temporal/ visual cortex | 0.74 | 0.87 | 0.020 |
| Left lateral temporal/ visual cortex | 0.71 | 0.86 | NS[b] |
| Right medial temporal/ visual cortex | 0.76 | 0.83 | 0.083 |
| Left medial temporal/ visual cortex | 0.78 | 0.87 | NS |

[a] Mann-Whitney $t$-test
[b] NS = not significant

## 78 NEUROACTIVATION AND NEUROIMAGING WITH SPET

**Table 3.** Mean regional brain perfusion rates[a] in autistic subjects compared with controls

| Region of brain | Autism (n = 4) Mean (% of control) | Controls (n = 4) Mean |
|---|---|---|
| Right frontal | 105.9 (62%) | 171.4 |
| Left frontal | 102.0 (58%) | 177.4 |
| Midline frontal | 128.5 (60%) | 215.5 |
| Right basal ganglia | 132.4 (64%) | 206.9 |
| Left basal ganglia | 129.1 (63%) | 204.0 |
| Visual cortex | 155.6 (72%) | 216.4 |
| Right lateral temporal (RLT) cortex | 114.2 (60%) | 188.8 |
| Left lateral temporal (LLT) cortex | 107.9 (58%) | 185.6 |
| Right medial temporal (RMT) cortex | 116.7 (65%) | 180.8 |
| Left medial temporal (LMT) cortex | 118.5 (63%) | 187.9 |
| Cerebellum | 155.9 (65%) | 239.2 |

[a] Perfusion rate = [(counts/ROI)/$^{99m}$Tc-HMPAO dose MBq] × 100, where ROI is the region of interest. All values differ significantly between the two groups ($p \leq 0.02$, Mann-Whitney $t$-test)

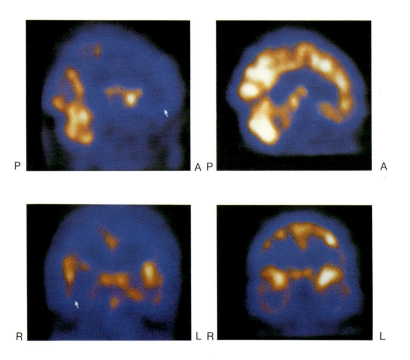

The global frontal and right temporal hypoperfusion that is found in the SPET images of autistic patients can be better understood by reviewing the previous functional neuroimaging studies in autism (Table 1). The first two PET studies in autism used $^{18}$FDG and found globally increased glucose metabolism in autistic subjects (A) versus controls (C) (A > C by 20% (Rumsey et al. 1985) and 12% (Horwitz et al. 1988)). In both studies subjects were sensory-deprived during a lengthy scanning protocol (150 minutes) requiring arterial cannulas and heating boxes over both hands. The same autism cohort was used in both studies, with 4 new autism subjects added in the second study. This cohort had a wide IQ range (verbal, <48 to 117; performance, <55 to 126). Autistic subjects who could not tolerate the lengthy scanning time, sensory-deprivation or arterial cannulas were excluded. Interestingly, the second study found decreased correlations of glucose utilization within and between the frontal and parietal lobes in the autism group (Horwitz et al. 1988).

In a PET study designed specifically to look for cerebellar abnormalities using $^{18}$FDG, 7 autistic subjects were studied while performing a continuous performance task (Heh et al. 1989). In this non-sensory-deprived state, no difference in glucose utilization was found between autistic subjects and controls. Unfortunately this study used only a single slice through the brain and did not afford the same regional comparisons as in other studies. Herold et al. (1988) used both $^{18}$FDG and $^{15}O_2$ steady-state inhalation and PET to study brain metabolism in autism. Their cohort of 6 autistic subjects differed from those in the previous studies in IQ and verbal skills. Additionally subjects were scanned in a relaxed atmosphere, listening to a tape of their favourite music. Herold et al. found no difference in $^{18}$FDG metabolism and no statistically significant difference in $^{15}O_2$ use between autistic subjects and controls. However, in all regions analysed the autistic subjects had lower $^{15}O_2$ metabolism than controls, although this was not statistically significant.

In summary, previous functional neuroimaging studies in autism have shown increased $^{18}$FDG metabolism in 14 patients, all of whom were sensory-deprived. A PET study using a different method ($^{15}O_2$ uptake), a different cohort and a different scanning environment revealed a trend towards hypometabolism that was not statistically significant. The one previous single photon study found globally decreased brain metabolism in autism. Thus, variables such as the cohort chosen, type of tracer used and the environment at the time of the scan are likely to influence the results of functional neuroimaging studies in autism.

◄ **Fig 17.** Sagittal (a) and coronal (b) HMPAO SPET scans of an adult patient with infantile autism (left) and a normal control (right). Note the decreased frontal and temporal perfusion in the autistic patient.

An important point that emerges from this review of functional neuroimaging in autism is that the environment and behaviour of the patient at the time of the ligand injection are absolutely critical. This vital point is often ignored when interpreting the results of single or cohort studies. The recent autism study at UCMSM differed from previous functional neuroimaging studies in terms of the environment at the time of scanning. The patients had their eyes open in a quiet room and were not sensory-deprived. This scanning environment more closely simulates the subjects' active resting state. Unlike the lengthy scanning times in PET, high-resolution SPET scanning takes only 15 minutes and does not require arterial cannulas or other anxiety-provoking invasive procedures, and can thus give a more 'life-like' picture of the functioning brain.

*Teaching Point*

> HMPAO SPET may play an important role in evaluating development disorders and mental retardation. Further studies are needed to determine whether this pattern of frontal and temporal hypometabolism is specific to autism and whether it correlates with age, IQ, mental retardation, scanning environment or other cohort variables. The environment and activity of the patient at the time of the rCBF ligand injection are very important to the interpretation of results of both scans of individual patients and group studies.

# Cerebrovascular Disease

SPET coupled with various ligands accurately represents and images rCBF. Thus the technique is particularly helpful in the area of cerebrovascular disease. Whether the change in flow is temporary (e.g. transient ischaemic attacks, migraine) or permanent (completed stroke), SPET can help in quantifying changes in cerebral blood flow.

## Stroke

The management of cerebrovascular disease by neurologists and other physicians has undergone several revolutions within the past few decades. The advent of CT scanning allowed physicians to localize cerebrovascular accidents (CVAs) as never before, and to determine whether they were ischaemic or haemorrhagic. Unfortunately, this revolution in properly diagnosing CVAs was not followed by similar advances in therapy. Functional neuroimaging with PET and SPET of the progression of CVAs has now given researchers a better understanding of the temporal profile of damaged neuronal tissue. Advances in stroke therapy appear imminent, and SPET should play a major role in assessing both the amount of damaged neuronal tissue and whether therapeutic measures are restoring blood flow in an appropriate manner.

## CASE 1

### Clinical Case History

This 74-year-old man had bilateral carotid stenosis with long-term claudication in his left leg. Recently he had been having symptoms suggestive of cholesterol emboli, with altered mental status.

DIAGNOSIS: Left cerebral hemisphere cerebrovascular accident (CVA)

### Image Acquisition Parameters

The patient was given intravenous 710 MBq $^{99m}$Tc-HMPAO. He was scanned supine on the GE/CGR Neurocam for 15 minutes (128 projections in a 64 × 64 matrix acquisition) using high-resolution collimators. Tomographic slices were reconstructed in the transaxial, coronal and sagittal planes using a Hanning prefilter with 1.0 cycles/cm cut-off frequency, a Ramp filter and attenuation correction (Fig. 18).

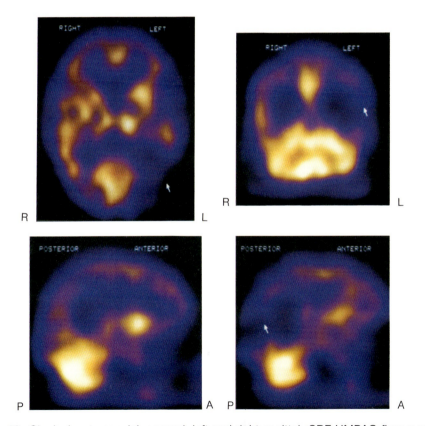

**Fig 18.** Clockwise, transaxial, coronal, left and right sagittal rCBF HMPAO flow maps confirm a single large perfusion deficit in the left parietal lobe consistent with an infarction.

## CASE 2

### Clinical Case History

This 72-year-old man had had a mild left brain CVA 10 years previously with mild right-sided body weakness. He had a carotid atheroma in his left carotid with a loud audible bruit, of which even he himself was aware. He was admitted for evaluation of a possible left carotid endarterectomy. He had hypertension, high cholesterol, and a positive family history of heart disease.

DIAGNOSIS: Carotid stenosis and atheroma

### Image Acquisition Parameters

The patient was given intravenous 680 MBq $^{99m}$Tc-HMPAO. He was scanned supine on the GE/CGR Neurocam for 15 minutes (128 projections in a 64 × 64 matrix acquisition) using general-purpose collimators. Tomographic slices were reconstructed in the transaxial, coronal and sagittal planes using a Hanning prefilter with 1.0 cycles/cm cut-off frequency, a Ramp filter and attenuation correction (Fig. 19). For the cerebral blood flow volume and cerebral reserve imaging see discussion on p. 86.

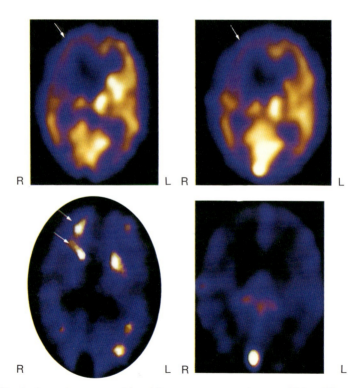

**Fig 19.** Clockwise, a transverse blood flow map, a superimposed blood flow and blood volume map, a blood volume-only map, and a cerebral perfusion reserve image (CBF/CBV) taken at the basal ganglia level are shown. There is impaired CBF and CBV in the right frontal lobe, but increased perfusion reserve. (See discussion on p. 86.)

## CASE 3

*Clinical Case History*

This 57-year-old man with hypertension had had several previous infarctions. On examination he was found to have a left homonymous hemianopia, impaired visuo-spatial skills, and weakness of his left arm and leg.

DIAGNOSIS: Multiple cerebral infarctions

*Image Acquisition Parameters*

The patient was given intravenous 760 MBq $^{99m}$Tc-HMPAO. He was scanned supine on the GE/CGR Neurocam for 15 minutes (128 projections in a 64 × 64 matrix acquisition) using high-resolution collimators. Tomographic slices were reconstructed in the transaxial, coronal and sagittal planes using a Hanning prefilter with 1.0 cycles/cm cut-off frequency, a Ramp filter and attenuation correction (Fig. 20).

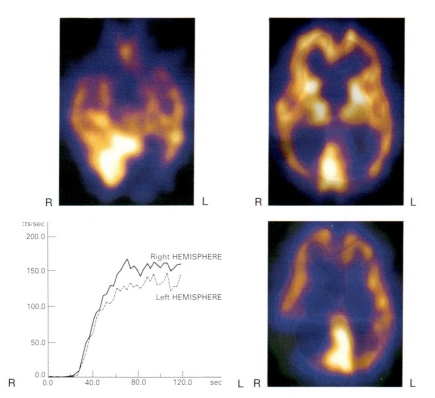

**Fig 20.** Clockwise, low, middle and high transverse flow maps, and time-activity curves obtained from regions of interest drawn over both hemispheres are shown. There are clear wedge-shaped perfusion deficits involving the left occipital and right parietal lobes. The cerebral time-activity curves confirm the asymmetry in uptake of the tracer due to carotid vessel disease.

## CASE 4

### Clinical Case History

This 39-year-old woman had a history of migraine headache since age 16, consisting of an aura over her right face and scalp. Two years before her scan she developed brief severe occipital headaches which were followed by left facial weakness lasting several hours. Since then she had had recurrent episodes of left facial drooping with left arm clumsiness lasting 2–3 hours and occurring 4–6 times per month. They were usually accompanied by an occipital headache. Multiple examinations consisting of CT, bilateral carotid and right vertebral angiography, echocardiography, CSF and serological examinations (including autoantibodies) and visual-evoked responses were unhelpful.

Examination between episodes was essentially normal. During the attacks she developed clear left facial weakness with mild left arm weakness.

DIAGNOSIS: Hemiplegic migraine

### Image Acquisition Parameters

The patient was given intravenous 720 MBq $^{99m}$Tc-HMPAO. She was scanned supine on the GE/CGR Neurocam for 15 minutes (128 projections in a 64 × 64 matrix acquisition) using high-resolution collimators. Tomographic slices were reconstructed in the transaxial, coronal and sagittal planes using a Hanning

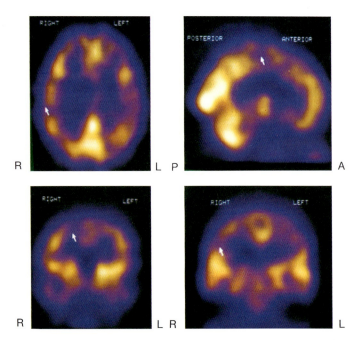

**Fig 21.** Clockwise, transaxial, paramedian right sagittal, and two anterior coronal flow maps. The arrows demonstrate a small area of impaired perfusion in the cortex possibly related to the patient's hemiplegic symptoms.

prefilter with 1.0 cycles/cm cut-off frequency, a Ramp filter and attenuation correction (Fig. 21).

## Comment

SPET neuroimaging has an important and expanding role to play in evaluating cerebral ischaemia associated with completed strokes and transient ischaemic attacks (TIAs). NeuroSPET has, or soon will have, a role to play in diagnosis, prognosis and evaluation of response to therapy (Holman and Tumeh 1990).

Most neurologists are unfortunately familiar with the clinical situation of a patient who presents with a new and unmistakable neurological deficit (for example, a left arm hemiplegia). An emergency CT scan is taken for diagnosis and to exclude a haemorrhage or subdural haematoma. Often this initial CT scan is normal. Structural imaging of ischaemic infarcts often lags several days behind the clinical progression, and thus it is sometimes several days before another CT scan can confirm the diagnosis. High-resolution neuroSPET can often aid a correct *and prompt* diagnosis. Rango et al. (1989) studied with SPET and CT 9 consecutive patients during the onset of their first-ever stroke. Decreased cortical rCBF on SPET in the appropriate brain regions was initially found in all patients. The initial CT scans were less sensitive than SPET in detecting ischaemic lesions. Thus SPET can aid an appropriate diagnosis in the early stages of stroke.

The second area of stroke management in which SPET may have a valuable role is in the prediction of future recovery. Structural imaging with CT shows an area of necrotic tissue at the centre of an ischaemic infarction; it does not show the surrounding area of tissue that has been damaged by ischaemia but which may recover (called the border zone of luxury perfusion). SPET on the other hand can often give an estimate of the extent of this peripheral damage at the edges of an acute infarct. Theoretically, the size of this border zone could be used to provide prognosis, or to dictate the amount of rehabilitation required. To test this hypothesis, Mountz et al. (1990) studied with CT and SPET 27 patients with cortical ischaemic infarcts. Patients were neurologically evaluated initially and at 1-year follow-up. The best predictor of neurological recovery was the log-transformation of the extent of initial SPET defect divided by the extent of damage on CT. The authors suggest that the relationship between the perfusion defects and tissue loss measured by SPET and CT have prognostic value following cortical strokes.

Finally, again capitalizing on SPET's ability to image the border zone surrounding acute infarcts, the technique might be used to judge the effectiveness of stroke therapies. Numerous medications are now under investigation for the acute treatment of cerebral ischaemia (calcium-channel blockers, vasodilators, free radical scavengers, excitatory amino acid inhibitors, etc.). These agents are currently studied in lengthy clinical trials in which subjects are given the experimental drug and then clinical response is evaluated months later. SPET scanning could theoretically play a role in judging the short-term effectiveness of these agents. An initial SPET scan, followed quickly by another after receiving the medication, may prove to be a quicker way of evaluating response, or of adjusting the dose to reduce the extent of the border zone.

The power of SPET in evaluating changes in blood flow after a therapeutic intervention was recently demonstrated in a study by Maurer et al. (1990). They used SPET and $^{123}$I-labelled amphetamine to study 20 patients before and after carotid endarterectomy. Using regional analysis they compared pre- and post-operative blood flow and found improvement in 79% of patients on the operated hemisphere, and in 42% of patients on the side opposite to their surgery.

Another interesting avenue of SPET research in cerebrovascular disease takes advantage of two routinely available radiopharmaceuticals: one, such as $^{99m}$Tc-HMPAO, to label rCBF and the other, such as $^{99m}$Tc-labelled autologous red cells, to label cerebral blood volume (rCBV). The relationship between rCBF and rCBV (rCBF/rCBV) has been explored and appears particularly promising as an indicator of circulation reserve. Good correlation between the rCBF/rCBV ratio and oxygen extraction in the brain has been demonstrated in normal volunteers and in patients with unilateral and bilateral carotid artery disease (Gibbs et al. 1984) (see also Fig. 19).

Using SPET it is possible to obtain in a single session, tomographic maps of the distribution of CBV and of CBF. A ratio image of rCBF/rCBV can then be obtained by computer manipulation (Sakai et al. 1985; Knapp et al. 1987). The methodology is simple and effective. In view of the close relationship which appears to exist between the rCBF/rCBV ratio and oxygen extraction, SPET therefore provides an indicator of metabolism. Despite its simplicity the method is not, however, without difficulties. While the flow map is relatively unambiguous (with counts per pixel of the order of 100–150), the volume map has a low count rate and produces a noisy image (with counts per pixel of the order of 5–20). There are thus difficulties with the reproducibility of the method and the correct definition of the anatomical boundaries of the blood volume map (most of the structures perceived on the flow image result from the large vessels and blood volume in the scalp).

The rCBV/rCBF method requires further technical validation and clinical evaluation but it holds promise. Work with this method has been applied to the investigation of dementia (Buell et al. 1990). More effort has been directed towards the evaluation of cerebrovascular disease (Buell et al. 1988) and of reserve before and after carotid surgery.

rCBF studies using $^{99m}$Tc-HMPAO have also been carried out to study paediatric cerebrovascular disease. Shahar et al. (1990) studied 15 infants and children with cerebrovascular disease ranging in age from 2 weeks to 16 years. All patients had a focal area of decreased rCBF. In 2 children SPET findings preceded abnormal CT findings, while in another 2, SPET was the only positive imaging test to correlate with focal clinical and EEG abnormalities.

SPET neuroimaging thus plays an important role in the management of cerebrovascular disease in both adults and children. It also offers exciting opportunities for improving management.

SPET is also being used to unravel several puzzling neuropsychiatric disorders long thought (but never proven) to be related to changes in blood flow. Stilhard et al. (1990) reported investigations in a patient whom they studied neuropsychologically and with $^{99m}$Tc-HMPAO SPET before and after an attack of transient global amnesia. The SPET scan during the attack showed severe bi-temporal hypoperfusion which returned to normal on a follow-up scan after the attack was over.

Many researchers have postulated that migraine headaches are caused by impaired cerebral autoregulation. SPET is beginning to unravel this complicated area. Studies using xenon-133 SPET in adults during migraine attacks have shown regional hypoperfusion in both classic migraine (preceded by an aura) and hemiplegic migraine (Oleson et al. 1981; Lauritzen et al. 1983). This regional hypoperfusion during attacks has been confirmed using $^{99m}$Tc-HMPAO in common migraine (without aura) and hemiplegic migraine (Podreka et al. 1987). Findings in migraine patients between attacks are less clear and more controversial, with most studies reporting an overall reduction in mean rCBF in migraine patients compared with controls (Levine et al. 1987; Podreka et al. 1987; Schlake et al. 1989). Battistella et al. (1990) studied 19 young migraineurs with $^{99m}$Tc-HMPAO SPET and found focally decreased rCBF in the temporo-occipital region (2 patients) and parietal region (2 patients). Those with SPET abnormalities had either classic migraine or hemiplegic migraine. Patients with common migraine had normal SPET scans between attacks.

*Teaching Point*

> HMPAO SPET scans accurately depict regional cerebral blood flow. In acute ischaemic strokes SPET is initially more sensitive than CT. Further, SPET helps identify damaged tissue that may recover with appropriate therapy. Thus, for any neuropsychiatric disorder thought to be due to changes in blood flow, SPET is both a powerful clinical and research tool. Multiple projections (not simply transaxial) may be needed to assess accurately the full extent of cerebrovascular disease.

# Major Psychiatric Illnesses

The field of psychiatry, unlike other branches of medicine, has long been hampered by an inability to study in detail the functioning human brain. Thus psychiatric researchers have either abandoned the brain altogether (behaviourists and strict psychotherapists), studied the brain peripherally (e.g. in terms of platelet function or CSF studies) or waited until the patient died for post-mortem analysis. SPET neuroimaging opens up a new world for psychiatry. This readily available and relatively inexpensive technology allows psychiatrists to look at the functioning brain in disease states. A brief overview of the initial findings in this burgeoning area is given below.

## Major Depression

### CASE 1

*Clinical Case History*

This 60-year-old man was in good health until 6 months before SPET scanning.

He gradually lost interest in his job, and had difficulty sleeping. He had decreased energy, which was worse in the morning, and a poor appetite. He was worried about his eventual retirement and poor financial state. He had frequent crying spells and intermittent thoughts of suicide. His mother had a history of depression. An evaluation by his general practitioner revealed a normal physical examination with normal baseline serologies and thyroid functions.

DIAGNOSIS: Major depressive episode

## Image Acquisition Parameters

The patient was given intravenous 760 MBq $^{99m}$Tc-HMPAO. He was scanned supine on the GE/CGR Neurocam for 15 minutes (128 projections in a 64 × 64 matrix acquisition) using high-resolution collimators. Tomographic slices were reconstructed in the transaxial, coronal and sagittal planes using a Hanning prefilter with 1.0 cycles/cm cut-off frequency, a Ramp filter and attenuation correction (Fig. 22).

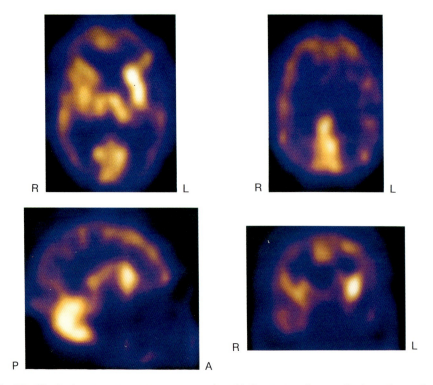

**Fig 22.** Clockwise, two transverse, coronal and left paramedian sagittal sections of an HMPAO blood flow study are shown. The findings are unexpected. There is reduced flow in most of the brain with the exception of the left caudate and putamen, which are normally perfused. An activation study carried out in this patient (see Chap. 10, p. 179) restores perfusion to the abnormal areas.

## CASE 2

### Clinical Case History

This 80-year-old woman had a 1-year history of worsening depression. She began to lose weight, and to lose interest in her daily activities. She experienced difficulty falling asleep and would frequently wake in the middle of the night and not be able to fall asleep again. She had a low mood with frequent crying spells. She displayed decreased motor movements and had slow thoughts and speech (psychomotor retardation). Her physical examination was non-focal and unremarkable. Serological studies and a cranial CT were normal.

DIAGNOSIS: Major depressive episode

### Image Acquisition Parameters

The patient was given intravenous 760 MBq $^{99m}$Tc-HMPAO. She was scanned supine on the GE/CGR Neurocam for 15 minutes (128 projections in a 64 × 64 matrix acquisition) using high-resolution collimators. Tomographic slices were reconstructed in the transaxial, coronal and sagittal planes using a Hanning prefilter with 1.0 cycles/cm cut-off frequency, a Ramp filter and attenuation correction (Fig. 23).

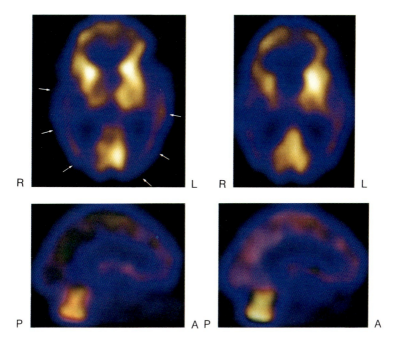

**Fig 23.** Clockwise, two transverse, left and right paramedian sagittal flow maps are shown. These are essentially normal with normal frontal perfusion. In a minority of cases of depression (~20%) SPET images are normal (see text). Both temporal lobes show impaired flow (arrows).

# CASE 3

## Clinical Case History

This 47-year-old woman had a long history of bipolar affective disorder. At age 19 she became severely depressed, requiring hospitalization. She had recurrent episodes of depression and two clear spells of mania. When manic she would go for several days without sleeping, and had pressured thoughts and speech with poor judgement. She had had no medication for two years before her scan. Six months before the scan she developed low mood with decreased energy and crying spells. There was a strong family history of depression. Her general examination was non-focal and a cranial CT scan was normal.

DIAGNOSIS: Bipolar-affective disorder, major depression

## Image Acquisition Parameters

The patient was given intravenous 700 MBq $^{99m}$Tc-HMPAO. She was scanned supine on the GE/CGR Neurocam for 15 minutes (128 projections in a 64 × 64 matrix acquisition) using high-resolution collimators. Tomographic slices were reconstructed in the transaxial, coronal and sagittal planes using a Hanning prefilter with 1.0 cycles/cm cut-off frequency, a Ramp filter and attenuation correction (Fig. 24).

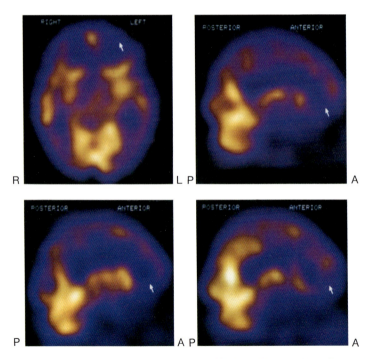

**Fig 24.** Clockwise, a transverse and selective right to left sagittal sections of cerebral blood flow maps are shown. The arrows point to decreased blood flow to the frontal lobe, frontal hypoperfusion frequently occurs in depression (see text).

## Comment

Major depression is a common disorder, affecting approximately 1 in 6 individuals at some point in their lives. The diagnosis has always been made on clinical grounds, but psychiatrists have looked for objective laboratory or clinical tests that could confirm the diagnosis and possibly predict response to treatment. Much excitement heralded the discovery of the dexamethasone suppression test (DST) in the 1970s. For the first time, modern psychiatry had a biological laboratory marker of an otherwise enigmatic disease.

SPET neuroimaging extends and confirms the DST in helping to make the diagnosis of major depression. SPET and PET studies have shown a consistent pattern of decreased frontal lobe activity in patients with depression, which resolves with treatment (O'Connell et al. 1989; Schwartz et al. 1987). This makes SPET a useful tool in diagnosing and following the clinical course of patients with depression. It can be particularly helpful in evaluating an elderly patient who may appear slightly demented. A SPET scan showing decreased frontal flow (and not the bi-parietal pattern of Alzheimer's disease) can reinforce the absolute necessity of a well-documented trial of antidepressant medications.

Well-designed SPET studies establishing the sensitivity and specificity of rCBF SPET for diagnosing major depression are needed. Additional SPET studies of patients with bipolar illness are also likely to prove valuable both clinically and for research.

Some cases of depression are not idiopathic and coincide with concurrent medical illnesses. Studying these types of depression with functional neuroimaging is likely to yield information that may help in understanding idiopathic depression. Schwartz et al. (1990) recently used $^{99m}$Tc-HMPAO SPET to study patients with depression following a cerebrovascular accident (post-stroke depression). Depression rating scores correlated with the volume of the ischaemic lesion as measured by SPET. Similar functional neuroimaging studies with SPET in medical conditions with a high co-morbidity of depression (e.g. multiple sclerosis, Parkinson's disease) are likely to be extremely valuable.

## Teaching Point

> rCBF SPET scans of patients with depression characteristically show decreased perfusion in the frontal lobes that normalizes with treatment. Depression is often accompanied by a decline in cognitive abilities. SPET scans can help distinguish between the true dementias and depression.

## Schizophrenia

### CASE 1

*Clinical Case History*

This 27-year-old man was well until age 20 when he developed tuberculous meningitis for which he was treated with three medications for 1 year. Twelve months after his initial infection he developed moodiness and apathy. He stared vacantly and talked nonsense. Investigations at that time included a repeat CSF study, cranial CT scan and EEG, all of which were normal. His symptoms at the time of his scan included apathy, episodes of bizarre behaviour with cutting of his clothes, and psychosis.

DIAGNOSIS: Probable schizophrenia, possibly exacerbated by TB meningitis

## Image Acquisition Parameters

The patient was given intravenous 740 MBq $^{99m}$Tc-HMPAO. He was scanned supine on the GE/CGR Neurocam for 15 minutes (128 projections in a 64 × 64 matrix acquisition) using high-resolution collimators. Tomographic slices were reconstructed in the transaxial, coronal and sagittal planes using a Hanning prefilter with 1.0 cycles/cm cut-off frequency, a Ramp filter and attenuation correction (Fig. 25).

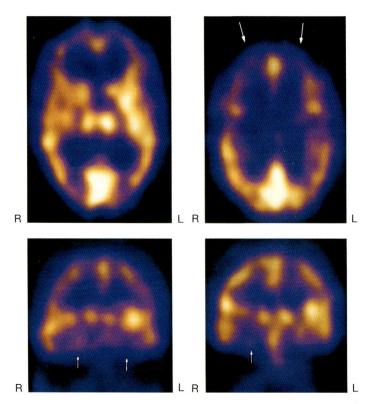

**Fig 25.** Clockwise, low and high transverse, and two midline coronal (posterior, anterior) flow maps are shown. In patients with schizophrenia rCBF SPET remains inconclusive. Occasionally, as in this case, bilateral medial temporal lobe low perfusion can be demonstrated, with normal lateral temporal lobe activity.

## Comment

rCBF SPET studies of patients with schizophrenia have shown conflicting and varying results with no clear picture yet emerging. Cohen et al. (1989) studied 10 chronically medicated schizophrenia patients and 5 controls using $^{123}$I-IMP. They found no differences in CBF compared with controls, although with their small control group there is a risk of a type II error. Some studies have shown increased bilateral caudate activity in patients with active psychosis. Other studies have shown decreased frontal and temporal activity compared with controls (Hawton et al. 1990; Paulman et al. 1990). As has been shown in other disease states, CBF hypoactivity often correlates with symptoms thought to originate from that part of the brain. For example, Paulman et al. (1990) found that decreased left frontal rCBF correlated with poor results on neuropsychological tests that involve the frontal lobes (Wisconsin Card Sorting Test, Luria-Nebraska Battery). A case study by Hawton et al. (1990) emphasized that the rCBF SPET patterns seen in schizophrenia are transient and often disappear with treatment.

Thus in schizophrenia, unlike the situation in Alzheimer's disease and depression, there is at present no characteristic or classical picture which uniformly helps with diagnosis. The rCBF SPET picture often corroborates the symptoms seen in schizophrenia, however, and may be used to monitor response to treatment. SPET may play a more important role in schizophrenia once the subgroups of the condition have been better understood, when better SPET ligands become more widely available, or when new and more effective treatments emerge.

There have been recent important advances in structural neuroimaging in schizophrenia which may have an effect on rCBF SPET. Recently Suddath et al. (1990) showed that in a group of monozygotic twins discordant for schizophrenia, quantitative MRI analysis of brain regions revealed significant decreases in temporal lobe volume in the schizophrenia group. This work remains to be expanded on with functional neuroimaging. Functional neuroimaging studies with rCBF SPET would be expected to reveal similar abnormalities in temporal and possibly frontal lobe functioning in schizophrenia. Unpublished work from our group at UCMSM shows temporal lobe hypoperfusion in rCBF SPET in patients with schizophrenia.

Another active and continuing area of SPET research in schizophrenia involves using specific D$_2$ ligands ($^{123}$I-IBZM: iodine-123-S(-)-N-[1-ethyl-2-pyrrolidinyl)methyl]-2-hydroxy-3-iodo-6-methoxybenzamide) (Kung et al. 1990) and SPET to study treatment response and possibly aid in diagnosis. This is discussed further in Chap. 10.

## Teaching Point

rCBF SPET scans of patients with active psychosis have shown increased activity in the basal ganglia bilaterally. The usefulness of this finding in diagnosing schizophrenia remains to be established. The recent structural abnormalities found with MRI in schizophrenia remain to be verified with rCBF SPET.

## Obsessive–Compulsive Disorder

### CASE 1

*Clinical Case History*

This 35-year-old man was well until age 25 when he began excessively cleaning his house after friends visited him. This compulsive urge to clean increased to the point where he spent several hours each day cleaning first his house and then himself. The behaviour became so severe that he could not entertain guests and several close friendships ended. He also lost his job because he was constantly delayed by the need to clean. He would often fall asleep at night in the bath, exhausted after several hours of compulsive ritualized cleaning. His general examination was normal.

DIAGNOSIS: Obsessive–compulsive disorder

*Image Acquisition Parameters*

The patient was given intravenous 720 MBq $^{99m}$Tc-HMPAO. He was scanned supine on the GE/CGR Neurocam for 15 minutes (128 projections in a 64 × 64

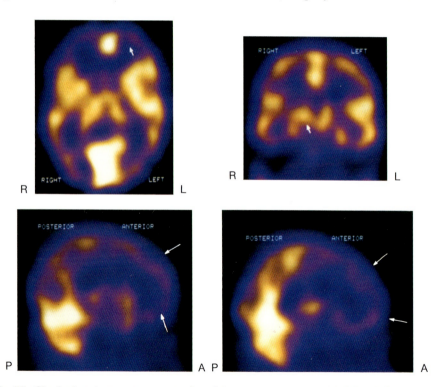

**Fig 26.** Clockwise, transverse, coronal and two paramedian sagittal blood flow maps. These demonstrate bilateral frontal hypoperfusion, even though this patient was not clinically depressed.

matrix acquisition) using high-resolution collimators. Tomographic slices were reconstructed in the transaxial, coronal and sagittal planes using a Hanning prefilter with 1.0 cycles/cm cut-off frequency, a Ramp filter and attenuation correction (Fig. 26).

## Comment

Some have referred to obsessive–compulsive disorder (OCD) as the neuropsychiatric disease of the 1980s and 1990s. For many years OCD patients suffered in silence as the condition was thought to be relatively uncommon and untreatable. Recently it has been found that OCD is common (occurring in 2%–3% of the population), is probably genetic, and can be treated by medications and behaviour therapy. The most interesting aspect of the disease, however, is that it appears to be clearly associated with dysfunction of discrete areas of the brain. All of these characteristics make the disease suitable for study with SPET neuroimaging.

Numerous case reports have shown that pathology of the orbital frontal and basal ganglia can sometimes cause OCD (for a review see George et al. 1991c). Frontal tumours (Brickner et al. 1940; Cambier et al. 1988; Seibyl et al. 1989) and infarctions of the frontal lobes and caudate nucleus can be the cause (McKeon et al. 1984; Tonkonogy and Barreira 1989; Weilburg et al. 1989). Similarly, infections involving the frontal lobes or basal ganglia are also known to produce OCD (Schilder 1938; Wohlfart et al. 1961; Laplane et al. 1981; Swedo et al. 1989b).

Further evidence of the role of the orbital frontal lobes and basal ganglia in OCD is provided by the results of psychosurgery. Surgically interrupting the frontally projecting fibres in the cingulum (a procedure known as cingulotomy) can often alleviate the symptoms of OCD (Talairach et al. 1973).

Previous functional neuroimaging studies of OCD have had conflicting results, with some demonstrating hypermetabolism (Baxter et al. 1988, 1990; Nordahl et al. 1989; Swedo et al. 1989a) and others hypometabolism (Laplane et al. 1989) of the frontal lobes. Three PET studies of OCD have shown similar but not identical results. Baxter et al. (1988) using $^{18}$FDG PET reported 10 OCD subjects with increased absolute metabolic rates in the heads of the caudate nuclei and orbital gyri when compared with controls. These findings were later replicated in a medication-free, age-matched and sex-matched controlled study with 10 OCD subjects. In this study the OCD subjects had increased metabolic rates in their orbital gyri when expressed as a ratio to the metabolic rate in the ipsilateral cerebral hemisphere. A PET study by Nordahl et al. (1989) revealed increased metabolic rates in the orbital gyri of 8 OCD subjects relative to the metabolic rate of the whole brain. Finally Swedo et al. (1989b) described 18 childhood-onset OCD subjects scanned with age-matched and sex-matched controls. These OCD subjects had abnormalities in the prefrontal and basal ganglia with elevated glucose metabolism in the left orbital frontal, right sensory-motor, and bilateral prefrontal and anterior cingulate regions. The right prefrontal and left anterior cingulate regions showed increased relative glucose metabolism. Additionally, a significant positive correlation emerged between glucose metabolic rate in the right orbital region and severity of the OCD.

In contrast, Laplane et al. (1989) reported on 8 OCD patients with bilateral lesions of the basal ganglia and a frontal-lobe-like syndrome. $^{18}$FDG PET scans in 7 patients revealed hypometabolism of the prefrontal cortex relative to other parts of the brain. These studies suggest that damage to the lentiform nuclei causes prefrontal cortex dysfunction which results in OCD. Additionally, there has been one case report of decreased activity in the right basal ganglia and anterior right temporal lobe in OCD using $^{123}$I-labelled amphetamine SPET scanning (Hamlin et al. 1989). These abnormalities resolved with pharmacological treatment. A recent study of OCD patients with concurrent Gilles de la Tourette syndrome (GTS) using $^{99m}$Tc-HMPAO found that OCD patients had decreased frontal activity and increased activity in the basal ganglia compared with subjects with simple GTS (George et al. 1991b).

*Teaching Point*

No clear picture has emerged of what rCBF SPET neuroimaging is likely to show in OCD, except that abnormalities of the frontal lobes and caudate nuclei (either increased or decreased activity) are common, and that the rCBF SPET images often normalize with treatment. SPET, with either rCBF or more specific dopamine or serotonin ligands, holds promise over the next few years to help unravel this fascinating disease.

# Movement Disorders

SPET imaging will undoubtedly play a large clinical role in the 1990s in the evaluation of patients with dementia, stroke and epilepsy. Following closely behind these areas in terms of the clinical impact of SPET is the interesting field of involuntary movement disorders. In many of these conditions structural neuroimaging is normal or unrevealing, as one wishes to know how the brain is functioning and not simply what it looks like structurally.

## Parkinson's Disease

### CASE 1

*Clinical Case History*

This 40-year-old man had a 1-year history of stiffness and clumsiness of his right arm with accompanying tremor. These symptoms responded well to treatment with dopamine. His symptoms at the time of his scan were mild (Hoehn and Yahr scale 1) and restricted to his right arm. His cranial CT scan was normal. He had no history of stroke-like episodes or head trauma. His family history was negative for movement disorders.

DIAGNOSIS: Right body hemi-Parkinson's disease

## Image Acquisition Parameters

The patient was given intravenous 720 MBq $^{99m}$Tc-HMPAO. He was scanned supine on the GE/CGR Neurocam for 15 minutes (128 projections in a 64 × 64 matrix acquisition) using high-resolution collimators. Tomographic slices were reconstructed in the transaxial, coronal and sagittal planes using a Hanning prefilter with 1.0 cycles/cm cut-off frequency, a Ramp filter and attenuation correction (Fig. 27).

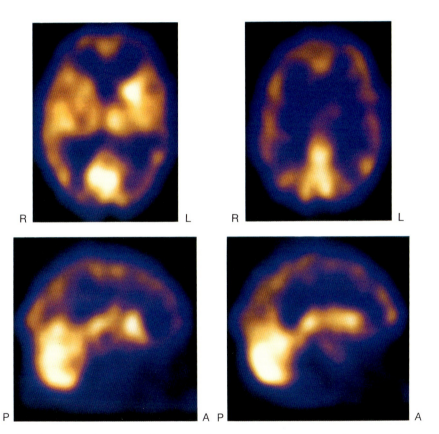

Fig 27. Clockwise, basal ganglia and high transverse, right and left parasagittal flow maps are shown. The SPET maps show asymmetry in blood flow to the caudate and thalamus. Blood flow studies are not diagnostic in early Parkinson's disease but may play a role in the future in the assessment of therapies, particularly when combined with more specific neuroligands (Chap. 2) or neuroactivation (Chap. 10).

## Comment

In idiopathic Parkinson's disease (PD) there is a loss of neuronal cells in the substantia nigra over time. This is thought to occur gradually throughout life, with symptoms manifesting only after 80% of dopaminergic cells in the substantia nigra are lost. General rCBF SPET scanning of PD patients often shows hypofrontality and decreased activity in the basal ganglia (Costa et al. 1988). As in the study of schizophrenia, much interesting SPET research in PD involves using specific $D_2$ binding ligands ($^{123}$I-IBZM) to image the dopamine system. If this ligand were widely available, $^{123}$I-IBZM SPET might possibly allow better diagnosis, and the prediction and evaluation of response to treatment in PD.

## Teaching Point

In general, rCBF SPET scanning of patients with Parkinson's disease shows decreased activity in the frontal lobes and basal ganglia. In cases where the disease is accompanied by a dementia, the rCBF SPET pattern can be more diffuse and resemble an Alzheimer's pattern, with parietal and temporal hypoperfusion.

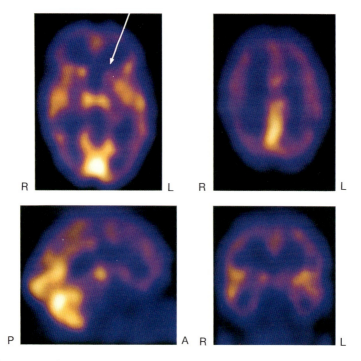

**Fig 28.** Clockwise, basal ganglia and high transverse, mid-temporal coronal and left parasagittal flow maps are shown. There are non-specific changes (mild). In patients with GTS, asymmetry of perfusion to the basal ganglia has been suspected, but more specific studies carried out with ligands such as dopamine-labelled tracers are likely to yield improved diagnosis of these patients.

# Gilles de la Tourette Syndrome

## CASE 1

*Clinical Case History*

This 35-year-old man first noticed mild facial twitches and tics at age 12. His tics would appear and last for several months, to be later replaced by a different tic or mannerism. He also noted intermittent sniffing, persistent coughing and an urge to repeat the last word of a sentence that someone had spoken (palilalia). Additionally he would constantly perform mathematical operations in his head and count things around him (arithromania). His mother was obsessively tidy and his uncle had mannerisms similar to the patient's. He came for diagnosis and treatment because of a complex tic that had occurred recently whereby he would have to move his hands violently up and down for several seconds to relieve tension. This interfered with his peformance at the bank where he worked. An EEG, CT scan and serological examinations were all negative.

DIAGNOSIS: Gilles de la Tourette syndrome

*Image Acquisition Parameters*

The patient was given intravenous 700 MBq $^{99m}$Tc-HMPAO. He was scanned supine on the GE/CGR Neurocam for 15 minutes (128 projections in a 64 × 64 matrix acquisition) using high-resolution collimators. Tomographic slices were reconstructed in the transaxial, coronal and sagittal planes using a Hanning prefilter with 1.0 cycles/cm cut-off frequency, a Ramp filter and attenuation correction (Fig. 28).

## CASE 2

*Clinical Case History*

This 14-year-old boy had begun to cough and sniff excessively at age 10. He would cough excessively for several months, then this would be replaced by sniffing. Additionally he had numerous blinking spells (blepharospasms) and jerks or twitches (tics) involving his head and neck. When entering rooms he was compelled to 'line up' objects and walk exactly through the centre of a door. If he did not do this properly, he would have to go back and re-enter the door. His father was noted to clear his throat excessively and had a mild facial tic. The boy's neurological examination, serology and cranial CT scan were all normal.

DIAGNOSIS: Gilles de la Tourette syndrome

*Image Acquisition Parameters*

The patient was given intravenous 10 MBq/kg $^{99m}$Tc-HMPAO. He was scanned supine on the GE/CGR Neurocam for 15 minutes (128 projections in a 64 × 64 matrix acquisition) using high-resolution collimators. Tomographic

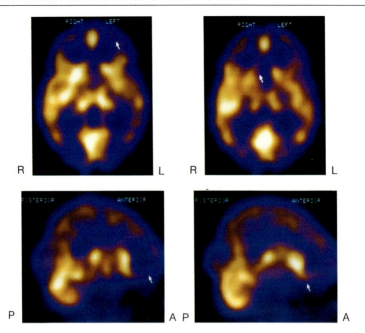

**Fig 29.** Clockwise, two transverse, right and left sagittal blood flow maps of GTS are shown. There is impairment of blood flow to both frontal lobes and mild asymmetry in the basal ganglia perfusion. The impaired frontal perfusion is consistent with the obsessive-compulsive symptoms.

slices were reconstructed in the transaxial, coronal and sagittal planes using a Hanning prefilter with 1.0 cycles/cm cut-off frequency, a Ramp filter and attenuation correction (Fig. 29).

## Comment

Gilles de la Tourette syndrome (GTS) is a complex neurobehavioural disorder characterized by fluctuating motor and vocal tics (quick motor movements/ twitches). GTS patients often have concurrent psychiatric problems such as obsessive–compulsive disorder, attention-deficit and hyperactivity disorder, and depression. Structural neuroimaging studies with CT and MRI have not found differences between GTS patients and controls. There is interesting new information emerging, however, that rCBF high-resolution SPET and specific $D_2$ SPET scans may be able to distinguish GTS patients from normals on a group basis (George et al. 1991b,d). SPET may also be used with activation techniques to help understand the origin (cortical or basal ganglia) of the tics in GTS.

## Teaching Point

rCBF SPET scans of patients with Gilles de la Tourette syndrome may show asymmetry or perfusion abnormalities of the basal ganglia. Specific $D_2$ ligands may improve SPET diagnosis of the syndrome.

# Huntington's Disease

## CASE 1

### Clinical Case History

A 71-year-old woman was noted by her husband to become progressively confused over the period of a year. On examination she demonstrated involuntary choreiform movements of her face and both arms. There was no family history of any similar disorder but it is known that both her parents died at a young age. Serological examinations were normal. A cranial CT was also unrevealing.

DIAGNOSIS: Huntington's disease (probable)

### Image Acquisition Parameters

The patient was given intravenous 710 MBq $^{99m}$Tc-HMPAO. She was scanned supine on the GE/CGR Neurocam for 15 minutes (128 projections in a 64 × 64 matrix acquisition) using high-resolution collimators. Tomographic slices were reconstructed in the transaxial, coronal and sagittal planes using a Hanning prefilter with 1.0 cycles/cm cut-off frequency, a Ramp filter and attenuation correction (Fig. 30).

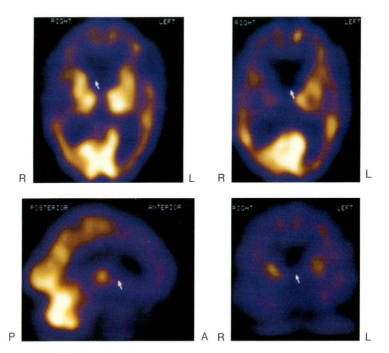

**Fig 30.** Clockwise, two transverse, a coronal and a right sagittal blood flow map are shown. The arrows point to the absence of perfusion in the basal ganglia in this patient with possible early Huntington's disease and a normal CT.

## Comment

Huntington's disease (HD) is a genetic neurodegenerative disease in which patients gradually develop chorea followed by dementia. Frequently other psychiatric disorders occur such as depression and impulsivity, and some patients have psychiatric symptoms as the first manifestion of their disease. Neuropathologically patients have gradual loss of the heads of the caudate nuclei, which can be seen using CT or MRI. A recent PET study of patients genetically at risk for HD found that functional neuroimaging with PET was a better predictor of the development of disease than was MRI or a detailed neurological examination (Mazziotta 1989). PET and rCBF SPET show decreased activity in the heads of the caudate nuclei bilaterally, giving in the axial view a characteristic 'pear-shaped' pattern to the ventricles. Further studies are needed to assess how sensitive and specific neuroSPET is for the diagnosis of HD.

## Teaching Point

rCBF SPET scans of patients with Huntington's disease show decreased perfusion in the heads of the caudate nuclei bilaterally. PET scanning has been proven in its ability to predict the development of Huntington's disease premorbidly. rCBF SPET is likely to replicate this finding.

## Sydenham's Chorea

### CASE 1

*Clinical Case History*

This 16-year-old right-handed girl presented to her neurologist complaining of involuntary movements of her left arm. A non-smoker who was not taking the contraceptive pill, she had a 1-year history of migraine, for which she took clonidine. Several weeks before her movements began she had a cold and sore throat with loss of her voice for several days. She first noticed variable twitching and jerking movements of her left arm, present daily, which would spread to involve the left side of her face and her left leg. She had difficulty walking and controlling her left arm while eating. Her birth and motor development were normal and there was no family history of movement disorders. Examination showed distinct choreiform movements of her left arm, hand and face, occasionally involving her left foot. She was otherwise normal with no heart murmur. CT scan, MRI, EEG and serological examinations were normal.

DIAGNOSIS: Probable Sydenham's chorea

*Image Acquisition Parameters*

The patient was given intravenous 10 MBq/kg $^{99m}$Tc-HMPAO. She was scanned supine on the GE/CGR Neurocam for 15 minutes (128 projections in a

64 × 64 matrix acquisition) using high-resolution collimators. Tomographic slices were reconstructed in the transaxial, coronal and sagittal planes using a Hanning prefilter with 1.0 cycles/cm cut-off frequency, a Ramp filter and attenuation correction (Fig. 31).

## Comment

Sydenham's chorea is a movement disorder which arises after a streptococcal infection. Usually several weeks after a throat infection the patient starts moving an arm or a leg involuntarily in a slow, twirling fashion (chorea). One theory of the aetiology of the movement disorder is that an autoimmune reaction starts at the time of the streptococcal infection and auto-antibodies are produced that mistakenly cross-react with neuronal cells in the basal ganglia. This damage is sufficient to cause neuronal damage and the movement disorder, but not large enough to be seen with MRI or CT.

There have been no functional imaging studies of Sydenham's chorea. But, as is apparent from this case, functional rCBF SPET imaging can help understand the underlying neuropathology, especially when structural neuroimaging is not revealing.

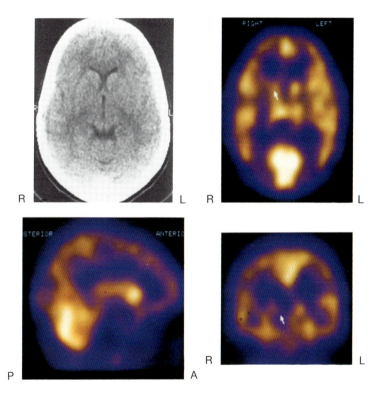

Fig 31. Clockwise, transverse CT and blood flow map, and coronal and right paramedian sagittal flow maps are shown. The arrows point to mild reduced perfusion in the right caudate nucleus, with normal flow elsewhere.

## Teaching Point

rCBF SPET scanning can aid in the diagnosis of movement disorders when structural neuroimaging with CT and MRI is non-revealing. Recent advances in SPET imaging have allowed shorter acquisition times (15 minutes), thus making it possible to image some patients with movement disorders.

## Fahr's Disease

### CASE 1

*Clinical Case History*

An 18-year-old boy presented with mild microcephaly, borderline mental retardation and a 5-year history of recurrent psychotic episodes. These

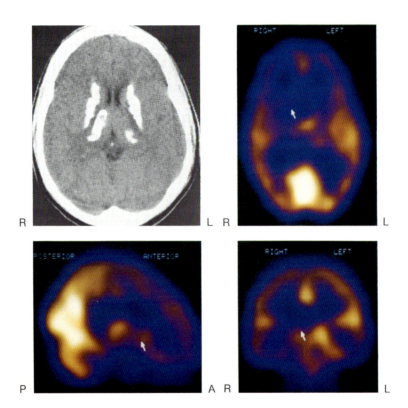

**Fig 32.** Clockwise, transverse CT and corresponding blood flow map, and mid-temporal coronal and right sagittal flow maps are shown. The CT demonstrates bilateral calcification in regions of the basal ganglia and surrounding tissue. The flow maps reveal low perfusion to the basal ganglia and the right frontal lobe.

episodes were characterized by auditory hallucinations and the delusional belief that he was the devil. These disturbances improved on treatment with phenothiazines. However, following the initiation of trifluoroperazine, a piperazine neuroleptic, he developed severe extrapyramidal side-effects of bradykinesia and cogwheel rigidity. When not receiving neuroleptics there were no abnormalities on neurological examination. In this patient metabolic calcium studies were normal and there was no relevant family history. A CT brain scan demonstrated significant bilateral calcification of the basal ganglia.

DIAGNOSIS: Fahr's disease (idiopathic basal ganglia calcification)

## Image Acquisition Parameters

The patient was given intravenous 710 MBq of $^{99m}$Tc-HMPAO. He was scanned supine on the GE/CGR Neurocam for 22 minutes (128 projections in a 64 × 64 matrix with 30-second acquisition) using high-resolution collimators. Tomographic slices were reconstructed in the transaxial, coronal and sagittal planes using a Hanning prefilter with 1.0 cycles/cm cut-off frequency, a Ramp filter and attenuation correction (Fig. 32).

## Comment

As the use of CT scans increases, idiopathic calcification of the vessels of the basal ganglia is noted with increasing frequency. In most cases this finding is thought to be of no clinical significance, and can be associated with aging. However, in a younger age group the calcification may be familial and associated with motor symptoms and intellectual deterioration. In some of these cases there may also be cerebellar calcification. It is interesting to note that in the case described above there was also a degree of decreased cerebellar uptake of $^{99m}$Tc-HMPAO.

Although not technically a movement disorder, Fahr's disease does involve the basal ganglia and is thus discussed here. There are very few published reports of functional neuroimaging of patients with calcification of the basal ganglia. Deisenhammer et al. (1989) reported that in two patients with Fahr's disease who received a SPET scan as part of an investigation into demented patients, there was no typical distribution pattern. Smith et al. (1988) reported that patients with Fahr's disease had varying degrees of underperfusion of the basal ganglia as demonstrated by an HMPAO scan.

## Teaching Point

This case highlights the importance of thinking about the brain as a series of interconnected regional areas (see Chap. 6). The basal ganglia and frontal lobes are inextricably linked.

The case also highlights the distinction between function and structure. Often rCBF SPET reveals functional changes even though the underlying brain structure as revealed by MRI or CT is intact. The opposite can also occur: a structural change such as calcification visible on CT does not necessarily imply a functional change visible on rCBF SPET.

# Malignancy

## CASE 1

### Clinical Case History

This 78-year-old man had developed cancer of the prostate 1 year previously. He underwent bilateral subcapsular orchidectomy. Four months later multiple bony metastases were noted on his chest radiograph. He did well on no therapy until 2 weeks before SPET scanning, when he noted unsteadiness, poor control of his right leg and a tremor and weakness of his right hand. A SPET scan was performed to help with his management.

DIAGNOSIS: Adenocarcinoma of the prostate with intracranial metastases

### Image Acquisition Parameters

The patient was given intravenous 710 MBq $^{99m}$Tc-HMPAO. He was scanned supine on the GE/CGR Neurocam for 15 minutes (128 projections in a 64 × 64 matrix acquisition) using high-resolution collimators. Tomographic slices were reconstructed in the transaxial, coronal and sagittal planes using a Hanning prefilter with 1.0 cycles/cm cut-off frequency, a Ramp filter and attenuation correction (Fig. 33).

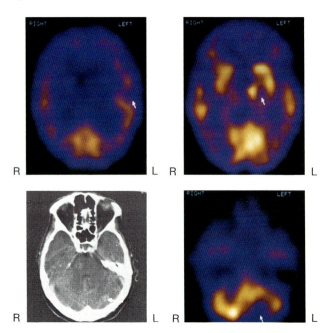

**Fig 33.** Three transverse cerebral blood flow maps and a transverse CT are shown. The SPET images reveal an appearance compatible with dilated ventricles, reduced blood flow to the frontal lobes, a possible left subcortical defect, but a definite abnormality in the left cerebellar hemisphere corresponding to the known malignancy.

## CASE 2

### Clinical Case History

This 79-year-old woman had developed weight loss 2 years previously accompanied by intermittent right facial pain. She was treated with carbamazepine which brought relief. One year before her scan she was noted to have non-tender hepatomegaly. Recently her facial pain had worsened. A cranial CT scan revealed a 2 cm enhancing lesion in the right middle temporal fossa. She had undergone a radical mastectomy with radiotherapy 25 years previously for carcinoma of the breast.

DIAGNOSIS: Carcinoma of the breast, with intracranial metastases

### Image Acquisition Parameters

The patient was given intravenous 10 MBq/kg $^{99m}$Tc-HMPAO. She was scanned supine on the GE/CGR Neurocam for 15 minutes (128 projections in a 64 × 64 matrix acquisition) using high-resolution collimators. Tomographic slices were reconstructed in the transaxial, coronal and sagittal planes using a Hanning prefilter with 1.0 cycles/cm cut-off frequency, a Ramp filter and attenuation correction (Fig. 34).

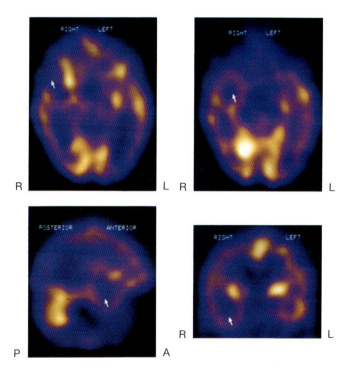

**Fig 34.** Clockwise, two transverse, mid-temporal coronal and right sagittal rCBF SPET flow maps are shown. The arrows point to an area of circumscribed perfusion abnormality in the right temporal lobe. On CT a 2 cm tumour was confirmed (not shown here).

## CASE 3

### Clinical Case History

This 54-year-old man was found to have a pinealoma in 1981. This was treated with radiation therapy and he had a ventriculo-peritoneal (VP) shunt placed to relieve an obstructive hydrocephalus. Recently he began to have episodes of decreased consciousness, loss of vision and ataxia. There was no evidence of a VP shunt blockage either clinically or radiographically. An abnormal CT scan showed no changes from previous images.

DIAGNOSIS: Vertebro-basilar insufficiency versus intermittent VP shunt blockage versus pinealoma recurrence

### Image Acquisition Parameters

For the rCBF study the patient was given intravenous 710 MBq $^{99m}$Tc-HMPAO. He was scanned supine on the GE/CGR Neurocam for 15 minutes (128 projections in a 64 × 64 matrix acquisition) using high-resolution collimators. Tomographic slices were reconstructed in the transaxial, coronal and sagittal planes using a Hanning prefilter with 1.0 cycles/cm cut-off frequency, a Ramp filter and attenuation correction (Fig. 35).

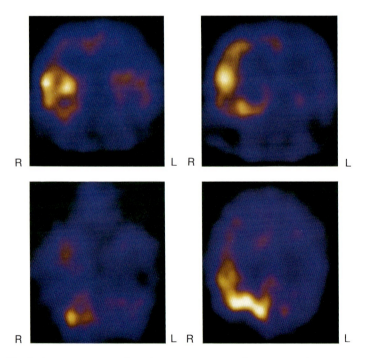

**Fig 35.** Clockwise, two coronal and two transverse flow maps demonstrate a large abnormality of flow mostly confined to the left hemisphere. The CT-demonstrated focal abnormality leads to wide-spread functional disturbance.

*Comment*

SPET neuroimaging can aid in the evaluation of CNS malignancies in two ways. First, using perfusion agents such as $^{99m}$Tc-HMPAO, SPET images show decreased perfusion in the areas of most CNS tumours. However, if the tumour is aggressive or excessively vascular, SPET rCBF agents will show hyperperfusion in those regions. Contralateral flow abnormalities are also seen in association with large tumours of the brain.

SPET has been used for many years to diagnose intracranial malignancy with conventional blood–brain barrier (BBB) tracers. Recent studies suggest that brain imaging with thallium-201 ($^{201}$Tl) more accurately reflects tumour grade. Kim et al. (1990) have reported the utility of a $^{201}$Tl index in distinguishing low-grade from high-grade gliomas. SPET can also help differentiate between tumour necrosis and recurrence of the tumour. Using a different tracer, L-3-[$^{123}$I]iodo-α-methyltyrosine, Langen et al. (1990) recently demonstrated increased uptake in 26 of 32 different tumours using SPET.

Thus SPET imaging with either conventional BBB flow agents, or agents such as thallium that collect in malignant tissue, can aid in the management of patients with CNS malignancies.

*Teaching Point*

> rCBF SPET studies of the blood–brain barrier can aid in the detection of large intracranial tumours when structural neuroimaging is not available. Also, SPET imaging with $^{201}$Tl used in conjunction with structural imaging can help estimate the grade of a malignancy. Finally, conventional rCBF SPET can be used to follow a patient after diagnosis to evaluate treatment response and distinguish between necrosis and recurrence.

# Epilepsy

SPET neuroimaging can be a useful clinical tool for physicians treating patients with epilepsy. It can be used to supplement an EEG for localizing the seizure focus – both at the time of the seizure (ictally) and between seizures (interictally).

## CASE 1

*Clinical Case History*

This 27-year-old man had suffered from multiple seizure types since childhood. At the time of his scan he had complex partial seizures, with occasional secondary generalization. These occurred approximately three times per month. He typically had an aura of an unpleasant sensation in his stomach followed by a foul odour. His general examination and a cranial CT scan were normal.

DIAGNOSIS: Complex partial epilepsy of probable temporal lobe origin

## Image Acquisition Parameters

The patient was given intravenous 680 MBq $^{99m}$Tc-HMPAO. He was scanned supine on the GE/CGR Neurocam for 15 minutes (128 projections in a 64 × 64 matrix acquisition) using high-resolution collimators. Tomographic slices were reconstructed in the transaxial, coronal and sagittal planes using a Hanning prefilter with 1.0 cycles/cm cut-off frequency, a Ramp filter and attenuation correction (Fig. 36).

## CASE 2

### Clinical Case History

This 20-year-old man presented with a 1-year history of intermittent twitching in his left leg. In addition he had suffered a seizure 6 months after the onset of this twitching, which started with jerking in the left leg and then rapidly progressed to a generalized convulsion. On examination he was found to have stimulus-sensitive myoclonus of the left leg. Neither CT nor MRI scans demonstrated any abnormality. He had no family history of seizures and no history of head trauma.

DIAGNOSIS: Stimulus-sensitive myoclonus of the left leg

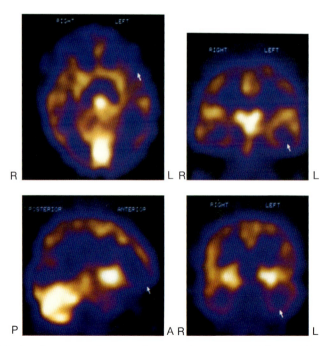

**Fig 36.** Clockwise, transverse, two mid-temporal coronal and left sagittal sections of the flow map are shown. The arrows point to a focal hypoperfusion abnormality in the left temporal lobe possibly related to the epileptogenic focus. The arrow on the sagittal section points to focal frontal hypoperfusion in this patient with concurrent depression.

## Image Acquisition Parameters

The patient was given intravenous 710 MBq $^{99m}$Tc-HMPAO. He was scanned supine on the GE/CGR Neurocam for 15 minutes (128 projections in a 64 × 64 matrix acquisition) using high-resolution collimators. Tomographic slices were reconstructed in the transaxial, coronal and sagittal planes using a Hanning prefilter with 1.0 cycles/cm cut-off frequency, a Ramp filter and attenuation correction (Fig. 37).

## CASE 3

### Clinical Case History

This 24-year-old man had had epilepsy since infancy with multiple different seizure types. At the time of his scan he was having focal seizures which occurred approximately 3–4 times per month. These would begin with a feeling of despair and depression, after which he could remember nothing. They occasionally spread and involved the whole body in a generalized convulsion. He was taking carbamazepine with no side effects. His general physical examination was unremarkable.

DIAGNOSIS: Complex partial epilepsy of probable temporal lobe origin

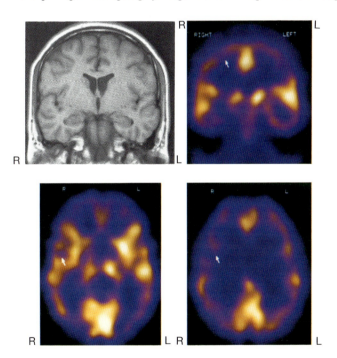

**Fig 37.** Clockwise, coronal MRI and corresponding flow map (interictal), and two transverse flow maps are shown. The arrows point to a region of focal hypoperfusion in the right motor strip possibly relating to the epileptic focus. This case is also presented in Chap. 10 (p. 177) where an activation study confirmed the suspected pathology.

## Image Acquisition Parameters

The patient was given intravenous 660 MBq $^{99m}$Tc-HMPAO. He was scanned supine on the GE/CGR Neurocam for 15 minutes (128 projections in a 64 × 64 matrix acquisition) using high-resolution collimators. Tomographic slices were reconstructed in the transaxial, coronal and sagittal planes using a Hanning prefilter with 1.0 cycles/cm cut-off frequency, a Ramp filter and attenuation correction (Fig. 38).

## Comment

Most epileptologists distinguish between focal epilepsy and generalized epilepsy. The focal epilepsies are thought to arise from dysfunctional neuronal tissue in a specific portion of the CNS – often the cortex (temporal or frontal lobes). Seizures may remain confined to this dysfunctional brain area, or may spread to involve the entire brain (secondarily generalize). In contrast, the generalized epilepsies (or primary generalized) are thought to stem from a diffuse dysfunction in neuronal tissue and to involve the entire brain from the outset of the seizure. To date, rCBF SPET scanning has been more extensively used in studying and managing patients with focal epilepsies.

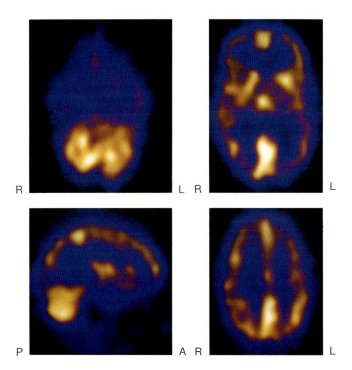

**Fig 38.** Clockwise, low, medium and high transverse and right sagittal sections of the flow map (interictal) are shown. There is symmetrical perfusion and no definite abnormalities were demonstrated. In this case of known focal epilepsy, the flow study was non-contributory.

Because focal seizures result from an electrical discharge in a discrete group of neurons, functional neuroimaging can help locate the origin of a focal seizure. PET studies first demonstrated a temporary rise in rCBF at the site of a focal seizure. Recent studies using rCBF SPET have confirmed the PET findings and have shown that rCBF SPET has an important role to play in the management of the focal epilepsies.

Shen et al. (1990) used $^{123}$I-HIPDM (iodine–123–$N,N,N$-trimethyl-n-[2-hydroxy-3-methyl-5-iodobenzyl]-1,3-propanediamine) and SPET to study 34 patients with focal epilepsy who eventually underwent temporal lobectomy for seizure control. In 93% of the subjects an ictal SPET scan showed focally increased rCBF at the seizure focus. Interictal SPET scanning of patients with focal epilepsy usually shows an area of hypoperfusion at the seizure site. In the study by Shen et al. (1990) 73% of patients had decreased regional cerebral perfusion at the seizure focus. Sixty-nine per cent of subjects showed both increased rCBF ictally and decreased rCBF interictally at the seizure focus – which was later surgically removed.

Duncan et al. (1990) studied 30 intractable epilepsy patients with CT, low-field MRI and SPET. rCBF SPET demonstrated lateralizing abnormalities in 19 of them, which is a much higher proportion than shown by CT (2/30) or MRI (15/30). Smith et al. (1989) studied 16 focal epilepsy patients with $^{99m}$Tc-HMPAO SPET. In those patients with good EEG localization, SPET imaging showed corresponding focal changes. In those patients with poor EEG localization, SPET scans failed to provide further information. Thus SPET can be a useful adjunct in the presurgical investigation of the patient with intractable focal epilepsy.

In other areas of epilepsy management, SPET sometimes gives important clinical information that EEGs and structural imaging fail to uncover. Katz et al. (1990) recently reported 2 patients with epilepsia partialis continua (constant focal seizures) in whom SPET imaging showed focal increases in rCBF in the appropriate brain region. In both cases the EEGs were entirely normal.

Finally, SPET has been used as a research tool for understanding the mechanisms behind the therapeutic effect of electroconvulsive therapy (ECT). Bajc et al. (1989) studied 11 patients undergoing ECT for the treatment of major depression. $^{99m}$Tc-HMPAO SPET scans were obtained 20 minutes after ECT, and 3 days later. Comparing the two scans of each patient, the authors found a relative increase in uptake in the frontal lobes (especially right side), fronto-temporal lobes and basal ganglia during the ictal scan.

## Associated Psychiatric Aspects of Epilepsy

### CASE 1

*Clinical Case History*

This 30-year-old man had had epilepsy since the age of 3. Born prematurely as a result of cephalopelvic disproportion, he suffered oxygen deprivation at birth and had left-sided seizures at age 2 days. Since then he has had multiple different seizure types. At the time of his scan he was having frequent (>3/day) attacks in which he would become atonic and fall to the ground. He had a 3-year history of command auditory hallucinations (voices telling him to perform certain actions) and obsessional behaviour. His medications were carbamazepine 400/500 and phenytoin 200/100.

DIAGNOSIS: Focal epilepsy, with secondary psychosis

## Image Acquisition Parameters

The patient was given intravenous 650 MBq $^{99m}$Tc-HMPAO. He was scanned supine on the GE/CGR Neurocam for 15 minutes (128 projections in a 64 × 64 matrix acquisition) using high-resolution collimators. Tomographic slices were reconstructed in the transaxial, coronal and sagittal planes using a Hanning prefilter with 1.0 cycles/cm cut-off frequency, a Ramp filter and attenuation correction (Fig. 39).

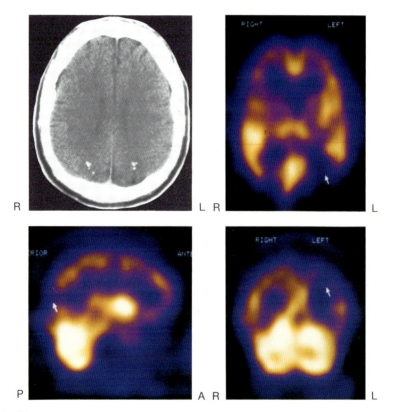

**Fig 39.** Clockwise, transverse CT and corresponding flow map, coronal and right paramedian sagittal flow maps are shown. Both the CT and SPET study demonstrate significant pathology in parietal lobes bilaterally, the arrow pointing to the larger of the two parietal flow abnormalities. The calcifications probably represent old trauma during seizures. Psychosis is sometimes associated with parietal lobe pathology (particularly right-sided).

## Comment

Epileptic patients sometimes have associated psychiatric symptoms such as paranoia, psychosis, or the 'Geschwind syndrome' of hypergraphia, hyper-religiosity and hyposexuality (Adams and Victor 1989; Trimble 1991). These patients can pose difficult management problems and SPET imaging can aid the understanding and treatment of these patients. Many view these psychiatric disturbances of epilepsy as useful models of the psychiatric symptom involved. SPET imaging, particularly using specific neurotransmitter ligands, should prove a useful tool in advancing this interesting field.

## Teaching Point

> Interictal rCBF SPET imaging in focal epilepsy often reveals an area of reduced flow at the seizure site. The area of abnormal flow is usually larger than the corresponding area of gliosis demonstrated by MRI. Ictal studies usually show focal areas of increased rCBF at the seizure site. When serial studies are undertaken in a patient with focal epilepsy the rCBF pattern clearly changes over time. A literature review gives estimates of 70%–90% accuracy for rCBF SPET in interictal localization of the site of a focal seizure. Despite these promising estimates, a definite assessment of the value of rCBF SPET as an accurate tool for localizing and lateralizing the site of focal epilepsies is yet to be determined. The role of rCBF SPET studies in an individual patient with a focal epilepsy also remains to be validated.

# Multiple Sclerosis

## CASE 1

### Clinical Case History

This 35-year-old woman had been in good health until age 25 when she had an attack of blurred vision which lasted for 2 months and then resolved. At age 27 she developed acute tingling and weakness in her left arm, which again resolved over time. A cranial MRI scan revealed multiple periventricular white matter lesions. Her CSF had oligoclonal bands and an increased IgG index. She was intermittently treated with high-dose steroids when her symptoms exacerbated. At the time of her scan she had a low mood and noted that her memory was poor. On examination she was found to have ataxia and slurred speech.

DIAGNOSIS: Multiple sclerosis

### Image Acquisition Parameters

The patient was given intravenous 700 MBq $^{99m}$Tc-HMPAO. She was scanned supine on the GE/CGR Neurocam for 15 minutes (128 projections in a 64 × 64 matrix acquisition) using high-resolution collimators. Tomographic slices were reconstructed in the transaxial, coronal and sagittal planes using a Hanning prefilter with 1.0 cycles/cm cut-off frequency, a Ramp filter and attenuation correction (Fig. 40).

## Comment

There is little published information in this area. One would expect multiple sclerosis (MS) plaques, in that they are damaged and necrotic tissue, to behave in SPET images much like infarcts. rCBF SPET imaging might prove a useful adjunct to MRI for judging the age and extent of MS lesions. However, MS plaques involve myelinated tissue (white matter) and are usually relatively small. rCBF SPET demonstrates grey matter lesions much better than it does white matter lesions, and this may limit the clinical role of rCBF SPET in MS.

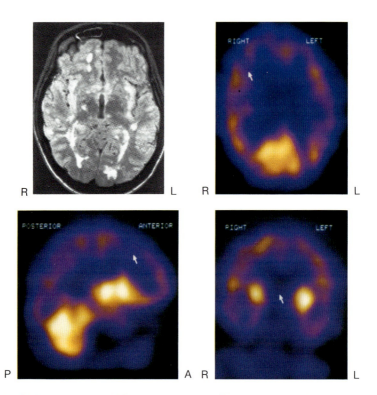

**Fig 40.** Clockwise, transverse MRI with corresponding flow map, mid-temporal coronal and left sagittal sections of the flow map are shown. The MRI demonstrates multiple white matter lesions, periventricularly and frontally, consistent with MS plaques. Flow maps in general are insensitive to white matter abnormalities. In this case, however, the SPET study shows the extent of perfusion abnormality in the white matter leading to a false appearance of enlarged ventricles (pseudo-hydrocephalus). (MRI scanner donated by the MS Society of Great Britain and Northern Ireland. Published courtesy of the MRI Research Group, Institute of Neurology, London.)

*Teaching Point*

rCBF SPET is much better at demonstrating lesions in grey matter than in white matter. The role of rCBF SPET in evaluating white matter diseases such as multiple sclerosis remains to be clarified.

## Conclusion

SPET imaging is a useful clinical tool which should improve patient care in neurology and psychiatry over the next few years. The preceding examples provide an overview of the ways in which rCBF SPET neuroimaging can aid in patient management. Clearly much work needs to be done to establish the sensitivity and specificity of SPET in detecting and evaluating various neuropsychiatric diseases. The new high-resolution SPET instruments allow for greater functional localization than ever before. Important as SPET is and will be in understanding brain function in various diseases, it also offers the exciting possibility of displaying the functioning healthy brain. Because of its versatility and widespread availability, SPET neuroimaging holds out the promise of allowing large numbers of researchers to investigate and understand brain organization and function. That aspect of SPET is considered in the second half of this book.

## References

Adams RJ, Victor M (1986) The principles of neurology. McGraw-Hill, New York
Bajc M, Medved V, Basic M et al. (1989) Acute effect of electroconvulsive therapy on brain perfusion assessed by $^{99m}$Tc-hexamethylpropylene-amineoxime and single photon emission tomography. Acta Psychiatr Scand 80:421–426
Battistella PA, Ruffilli R, Pozza FD et al. (1990) $^{99}$Tc-HMPAO SPET in pediatric migraine. Headache 30:646–649
Baxter LR, Schwartz JM, Mazziotta JC et al. (1988) Cerebral glucose metabolic rates in non-depressed patients with obsessive–compulsive disorder. Am J Psychiatry 145:1560–1563
Baxter LR, Schwartz JM, Guze BH, Bergman K, Szuba MP (1990) PET imaging in obsessive compulsive disorder with and without depression. J Clin Psychiatry 51:61–69
Brickner RM, Rosner AA, Munro R (1940) Physiological aspects of the obsessive state. Psychosom Med 2:369–383
Buell U, Braun H, Ferbert A et al. (1988) Combined SPECT imaging of regional cerebral blood flow and blood volume to assess regional cerebral perfusion reserve in patients with cerebrovascular disease. Nucl Med 27:51–56
Buell U, Reiche W, Weiller C et al. (1990) Binswanger's disease (BD): results of brain SPET (flow-volume) compared to MRI. Eur J Nucl Med 16:419 (abstr)
Burns A, Philpott MP, Costa DC et al. (1989) The investigation of Alzheimer's disease with single photon emission tomography. J Neurol Neurosurg Psychiatry 52:248–253
Cambier J. Masson C, Benammou S, Robine B (1988) La graphomanie, activité graphique compulsive manifestation d'un gliome fronto-calleux. Rev Neur 144:158–164
Cohen MB, Lake RR, Graham LS et al. (1989) Quantitative iodine-123 IMP imaging of brain perfusion in schizophrenia. J Nucl Med 30:1616–1620
Costa DC, Ell RJ, Burns A, Philpot M, Levy R (1988) rCBF tomograms and Tc-HMPAO in patients

with dementia (Alzheimer's type and HIV) and Parkinson's disease: initial results. J Cereb Blood Flow 8:109–115

Courchesne E, Yeung-Courchesne R, Press GA, Hesselink JR, Jernigan TL (1988) Hypoplasia of cerebellar vermal lobules VI and VII in autism. N Engl J Med 318:1349–1354

Deisenhammer E, Reisecker F, Leblhuber F, Holl K, Markut H, Trenkler J, Schneider I (1989) Single photon emission-computed tomography in the differential diagnosis of dementia. Dtsch Med Wochenschr 114:1639–1644

Denays R, Tondeur M, Foulon M et al. (1989) Regional brain blood flow in congenital dysphasia: studies with technetium-99m-HMPAO SPECT. J Nucl Med 30:1825–1829

Denays R, Tondeur M, Toppet V et al. (1990) Cerebral palsy: initial experience with Tc-99m HMPAO SPECT of the brain. Radiology 175:111–116

Duncan R, Patterson J, Hadley DM et al. (1990) CT, MR and SPECT imaging in temporal lobe epilepsy. J Neurol Neurosurg Psychiatry 53:11–15

Ell PJ, Cullum I, Costa DC (1985) Regional cerebral blood flow mapping with a new Tc-99m-labelled compound. Lancet ii:50–51

Gaffney GR, Kuperman S, Tsai LY, Minchin S (1989) Forebrain structures in infantile autism. J Am Acad Child Adolesc Psychiatry 28:534–537

Gemmell HG, Sharp PF, Besson JA et al. (1987) Differential diagnosis in dementia using the cerebral blood flow agent $^{99m}$Tc-HMPAO: a SPECT study. J Comput Assist Tomogr 11:398–402

George MS, Costa DC, Kouris K, Ring H, Ell PJ (1991a) $^{99}$Tc$^{m}$-HMPAO abnormalities in infantile autism. Proceedings of the American Psychiatric Association Annual Meeting (abstr) (in press)

George MS, Robertson MM, Costa DC, Trimble MR, Ell PJ (1991b) HMPAO SPECT scans of co-morbid OCD/GTS patients. Proceedings of the American Psychiatric Association Annual Meeting (abstr) (in press)

George MS, Melvin JA, Kellner CH (1991c) Obsessive-compulsive symptoms in neurologic disease. Beh Neurol (in press)

George MS, Robertson MM, Costa DC, Ell PJ (1991d) $D_2$ receptor activity in Tourette syndrome (GTS). Proceedings of the American Psychiatric Association Annual Meeting (abstr) (in press)

Gibbs JM, Wise RJS, Lenders KL, Jones T (1984) Evaluation of cerebral perfusion reserve in patients with carotid-artery occlusion. Lancet ii:310–314

Hamlin CL, Swayne LC, Liebowitz MR (1989) Striatal IMP-SPECT decrease in obsessive-compulsive disorder, normalized by pharmacotherapy. Neuropsychia, Neuropsychol Beh Neurol 2:290–300

Hashimoto T, Tayama M, Mori K, Fujino K, Miyazaki M, Kuroda Y (1989) Magnetic resonance imaging in autism: preliminary report. Neuropediatrics 20:143–146

Hawton K, Shepstone B, Soper N, Reznek L (1990) Single-photon emission computerized tomography (SPECT) in schizophrenia. Br J Psychiatry 156:425–427

Heh CW, Smith R, Wu J et al. (1989) Positron emission tomography of the cerebellum in autism. Am J Psychiatry 146:242–245

Herold S, Frackowiak RS, Le Couteur A, Rutter M, Howlin P (1988) Cerebral blood flow and metabolism of oxygen and glucose in young autistic adults. Psychol Med 18:823–831

Holman BL (1986) Perfusion and receptor SPECT in the dementias. J Nucl Med 27:855–860

Holman BL, Tumeh SS (1990) Single-photon emission computed tomography (SPECT). JAMA 263:561–564

Horwitz B, Rumsey JM, Grady CL, Rapoport SI (1988) The cerebral metabolic landscape in autism: intercorrelations of regional glucose utilization. Arch Neurol 45:749–755

Johnson KA, Holman BL, Rosen TJ, Nagel JS, English RJ, Growdon JH (1991) I-123 IMP SPECT is accurate in the diagnosis of Alzheimer's disease. Arch Intern Med (in press)

Katz A, Bose A, Lind SJ, Spencer SS (1990) SPECT in patients with epilepsia partialis continua. Neurology 40:1848–1850

Kim KT, Black KL, Marciano D et al. (1990) Thallium-201 SPECT imaging of brain tumors: methods and results. J Nucl Med 31:965–969

Knapp WH, Kummer R, Kubler W (1986) Imaging of cerebral blood flow-to-volume distribution using SPECT. J Nucl Med 27: 465–470

Kung HF, Alavi A, Chang W et al. (1990) In vivo SPECT imaging of CNS D-2 dopamine receptors: initial studies with iodine-123-IBZM in humans. J Nucl Med 31:573–579

Langen KJ, Coenen HH, Roosen N et al. (1990) SPECT studies of brain tumors with L-3-[$^{123}$I]iodo-alpha-methyl tyrosine: comparison with PET, $^{124}$IMT and first clinical results. J Nucl Med 31:281–286

Laplane D, Widlocher D, Pillon B, Baulac M, Binoux F (1981) Comportement compulsif d'allure obsessionnelle par necrose circonscrite bilaterale pallido-striatale. Rev Neurol 137:269–276

Laplane D, Levasseur M, Pillon B et al. (1989) Obsessive–compulsive and other behavioural changes with bilateral basal ganglia lesions. Brain 112:699–725

Lauritzen M, Olsen TS, Lassen NA, Paulson OB (1983) Changes in regional cerebral blood flow during the course of classic migraine attacks. Ann Neurol 13:633–641

Levine SR, Welch KMA, Ewing JR, Robertson WM (1987) Asymmetric cerebral blood flow patterns in migraine. Cephalagia 7:245–248

Lou HC, Henriksen L, Bruhn P (1990) Focal cerebral dysfunction in developmental learning disabilities. Lancet 335:8–11

Mazziotta JC (1989) Huntington's disease: studies with structural imaging techniques and positron emission tomography. Semin Neurol 9:360–369

Maurer AH, Siegel JA, Comerota AJ, Morgan WA, Johnson MH (1990) SPECT quantification of cerebral ischemia before and after carotid endarterectomy. J Nucl Med 31:1412–1420

McKeon J, McGuffin P, Robinson P (1984) Obsessive–compulsive neurosis following head injury: a report of four cases. Br J Psychiatry 144:190–192

Montaldi D, Brooks DN, McColl JH et al. (1990) Measurements of regional cerebral blood flow and cognitive performance in Alzheimer's disease. J Neurol Neurosurg Psychiatry 53:33–38

Mountz JM, Modell JG, Foster NL et al. (1990) Prognostication of recovery following stroke using the comparison of CT and technetium-99m HM-PAO SPECT. J Nucl Med 31:61–66

Murakami JW, Courchesne E, Press GA, Yeung-Courchesne R, Hesselink JR (1989) Reduced cerebellar hemisphere size and its relationship to vermal hypoplasia. Arch Neurol 46:689–694

Neary D, Snowden JS, Mann DMA, Northen B, Goulding JP, Macdermott N (1990) Frontal lobe dementia and motor neuron disease. J Neurol Neurosurg Psychiatry 53:23–32

Nordahl TE, Benkelfat C, Semple WE et al. (1989) Cerebral glucose metabolic rates in obsessive–compulsive disorder. Neuropsychopharmacology 2:23–28 (abstr)

O'Connel RA, Van Heertum RL, Billick SB, Holt AR, Gonzalez A, Notardonato H, Luck D, King LN (1989) Single photon emission computed tomography (SPECT) with IMP in the differential diagnosis of psychiatric disorders. J Neuropsychiatry 1:145–153

Oleson J, Larsen B, Lauritzen M (1981) Focal hyperemia followed by spreading oligemia and impaired activation of rCBF in classic migraine. Ann Neurol 9:344–352

Paulman RG, Devous MD, Gregory RR et al. (1990) Hypofrontality and cognitive impairment in schizophrenia: dynamic single-photon tomography and neuropsychological assessment of schizophrenic brain function. Biol Psychiatry 27:377–399

Penfield W, Rasmussen T (1950) The cerebral cortex of man. Macmillan, New York

Piven J, Berthier ML, Starkstein SE, Nehme E, Pearlson G, Folstein S (1990) Magnetic resonance imaging evidence for a defect of cerebral cortical development in autism. Am J Psychiatry 147:734–739

Plioplys AV, Hemmens SE, Regan CM (1990) Expression of a neural cell adhesion molecule serum fragment is depressed in autism. J Neuropsychiatry 2:413–417

Podreka I, Suess E, Goldenberg G et al. (1987) Initial experience with technetium-99m-HM-PAO brain SPECT. J Nucl Med 28:1657–1666

Rango M, Candelise L, Perani D et al. (1989) Cortical pathophysiology and clinical neurologic abnormalities in acute cerebral ischemia. A serial study with single photon emission computed tomography. Arch Neurol 46:1318–1322

Reed BR, Jagust WJ, Seab JP, Ober BA (1989) Memory and regional cerebral blood flow in mildly symptomatic Alzheimer's disease. Neurology 39:1537–1539

Rubinstein M, Denays R, Ham HR (1989) Functional imaging of brain maturation in humans using iodine-123-iodoamphetamine and SPECT. J Nucl Med 30:1982–1985

Rumsey JM, Duara R, Grady C et al. (1985) Brain metabolism in autism. Resting cerebral glucose utilization rates as measured with positron emission tomography. Arch Gen Psych 42:488–455

Sakai F, Nakazawa K, Tazaki Y et al. (1985) Regional cerebral blood volume and hematocrit measured in normal human volunteers by SPECT. J Cerebr Blood Flow Metab 5:207–213

Schilder P (1938) The organic background of obsessions and compulsions. Am J Psychiatry 95:1397–1413

Schlake HP, Bottger IG, Grotemeyer KH, Husstedt IW (1989) Brain imaging with $^{123}$I-IMP SPECT in migraine between attacks. Headache 29:344–349

Schwartz JM, Speed NM, Mountz JM, Gross MD, Modell JG, Kuhl DE (1990) $^{99m}$Tc-hexamethyl-propyleneamine oxime single photon emission CT in poststroke depression. Am J Psychiatry 147:242–244

Schwartz JM, Baxter LR, Mazziotta JC et al. (1987) The differential diagnosis of depression: relevance of positron emission tomography studies of cerebral glucose metabolism to the bipolar–unipolar dichotomy. JAMA 258:1368–1374

Seibyl JP, Krystal JH, Goodman WK, Price LH (1989) Obsessive–compulsive symptoms in a patient with a right frontal lobe lesion. Neuropsychia, Neuropsychol Beh Neurol 1:295–299

Shahar E, Gilday DL, Hwang PA, Cohen EK, Lambert R (1990) Pediatric cerebrovascular disease: alterations of regional cerebral blood flow detected by $^{99m}$Tc-HMPAO SPECT. Arch Neurol 47:578–584

Shen W, Lee BI, Park HM et al. (1990) HIPDM-SPECT brain imaging in the presurgical evaluation of patients with intractable seizures. J Nucl Med 31:1280–1284

Sherman M, Nass R, Shapiro T (1984) Regional cerebral blood flow in infantile autism. J Autism Dev Dis 4:438–440

Smith DF, Smith FW, Knight RS, Roberts RC, Gemmell HG (1989) $^{99}$Tc$^{m}$-HMPAO single photon emission computed tomography in partial epilepsy: a preliminary report. Br J Radiol 62:970–973

Smith FW, Gemmell HG, Sharp PF, Besson JA (1988) Technetium-99m HMPAO imaging in patients with basal ganglia disease. Br J Radiol 61:914–920

Stilhard G, Landis T, Schiess R, Regard M, Sialer G (1990) Bitemporal hypoperfusion in transient global amnesia: $^{99m}$Tc-HM-PAO SPECT and neuropsychological findings during and after an attack. J Neurol Neurosurg Psychiatry 53:339–342

Stuss DT, Benson DF (1986) The frontal lobes. Raven Press, New York

Suddath RL, Christison GW, Torrey EF, Casanova M, Weinberger DR (1990) Anatomical abnormalities in the brains of monozygotic twins discordant for schizophrenia. N Engl J Med 322:789–794

Swedo SE, Schapiro MB, Grady CL (1989a) Cerebral glucose metabolism in childhood-onset obsessive–compulsive disorder. Arch Gen Psych 46:518–523

Swedo SE, Rapoport JL, Cheslow DL et al. (1989b) High prevalence of obsessive–compulsive symptoms in patients with Sydenham's chorea. Am J Psychiatry 146:246–249

Talairach J, Bancaud J, Geier S et al. (1973) The cingulate gyrus and human behaviour. Electroencephalogr Clin Neurol 34:45–52

Terry RD, Katzman R (1983) Senile dementia of the Alzheimer's type. Ann Neurol 14:497–506

Tonkonogy J, Barreira P (1989) Obsessive–compulsive disorder and caudate–frontal lesion. Neuropsychia, Neuropsychol Beh Neurol 2:203–209

Trimble MR (1991) The psychoses of epilepsy. Raven Press, New York

Weilburg JB, Mesulam M, Weintraub S, Buonanno F, Jenike M, Stakes JW (1989) Focal striatal abnormalities in a patient with obsessive–compulsive disorder. Arch Neurol 46:233–235

Wohlfart G, Ingvar DH, Hellberg A (1961) Compulsory shouting (Benedek's 'klazomania') associated with oculogyric spasms in chronic epidemic encephalitis. Acta Psychiatr Scand 36:369–377

*Part II:*
# Neuroactivation with SPET

# Chapter 5
# A Historical and Philosophical Review of Localizing Brain Function

Functional neuroimaging with SPET and PET can be viewed as the latest chapter in a long historical debate about how the mind interacts with the brain. This debate is a fundamental one for mankind, as we try to understand how we are able to perform those actions that most make us human – thinking, planning, dreaming, grieving. It is both interesting and entertaining to look back over this debate about how the brain and mind work. However, reviewing this history is more than simply an amusing historical game. For only by looking back and realizing how we arrived at our present theories of how the brain functions can we then proceed to ask the important questions that functional neuroimaging allows us to investigate.

## A Historical Review of Localization

Perhaps the first people to engage in functional neuroimaging were pre-literate shamans. Some pre-literate societies practised trephining: hollowing out a hole in the skull and viewing the brain in an alive patient. We can only speculate about their underlying notions of the brain and mind and why they were performing these operations. Remarkably some patients apparently survived trephining, performed without anaesthesia or antibiotics. Skulls have been found with bone growth around the edges of trephined holes, indicating that the patient lived for some time after the operation. Additionally, some skulls have been found with more than one hole. Clearly these shamans somehow felt that the brain, or at least the skull, had something to do with illness or magic, but that is all that we know.

Moving from prehistory to the Middle Ages, one of the most important figures in the history of Western medicine was Galen. Galen's concept of disease revolved around understanding the four bodily humours. All diseases were the result of an imbalance of the mixture of these four humours. Therapy was aimed at restoring the previous harmony by bloodletting, purgatives and cathartics. Although this is by design a systemic view of disease, some localization was incorporated into the Galenic theory. For example, headaches were thought to arise from bad humours in the ventricles of the brain. But generally speaking, the Galenic view of disease had very little room for localization of diseases or functions. Further understanding of specific local brain function could only occur after Galen's theories were replaced. This did not occur until fairly recently. The seventeenth century saw a renewal of interest in the brain as the location of many mental diseases. Several writers of this period outlined the beginnings of theories of cerebral localization. One of the founders of neurology as a discipline was Sir Thomas Willis. A student of William Harvey, who had pioneered the concepts of venous and arterial circulation, Willis largely rejected the teachings he had received concerning the humoral theory of disease (Hill and George 1987). Through keen clinical observation and autopsy studies Willis reforged his thinking about the brain and disease. In contrast to the Galenic teaching of his time, Willis argued that the substance of the brain had specific functions. Willis rethought the ideas concerning headache, arguing that the underlying cause of headache was in the brain substance, and not in the blood or gastrointestinal system as had been previously thought. Willis was clearly one of the first to reject the humoral theory and to begin to equate mental disease with altered brain function. Concepts of cerebral localization continued after Willis. The height of the revolution toward locating mental illness in the brain came with the writings of Gall and Spurzheim and the movement known as phrenology (Trimble 1988). According to the phrenologists, the human brain was composed of different organs, many of which could be palpated through the scalp (Fig. 1). Unfortunately, phrenology fell into disrepute when its practice was taken over by charlatans and non-medical practitioners. However, the zeal of the phrenologists for localization may be seen as a reactionary swing of the pendulum away from the non-localization theories of Galen and Descartes.

Much of established medicine in the early 1800s still held the view that mental functions could not be localized to specific brain regions. The concept of localization was resurrected, however, by Broca in 1861 who described eight patients with a loss of speech, all of whom had lesions in the third left frontal convolution (now known as Broca's area). At the same time, John Hughlings Jackson, David Ferrier and others were pioneering the concept of cerebral localization of certain diseases, most notably epilepsy. Jackson was perhaps the first to make an important distinction that directly impacts on modern functional neuroimaging. Jackson argued that while it may be possible to localize a lesion, it is much more difficult to localize a function. He also pioneered the concept of negative (ablative) versus positive (irritative) aspects of lesions and brain function. A lesion in the same part of the cortex might produce different symptoms, depending upon whether it destroyed tissue, or irritated neurons and caused them to carry out their normal functions in a pathological way. Most physicians who perform modern functional neuroimaging would do well to remember these two lessons from Jackson: (1) that lesions can be localized more easily than functions and (2) that lesions can be ablative (destructive) or irritative (an enhancement of normal function) (Taylor 1958).

Modern clinical neurology, with its emphasis on lesion localization, followed quickly on the heels of Jackson, Ferrier and others. But Jackson's distinction between positive symptoms and ablative symptoms seems to have been neglected. Much of modern neurology's understanding of the brain came from meticulously following patients with strokes and tumours to autopsy and

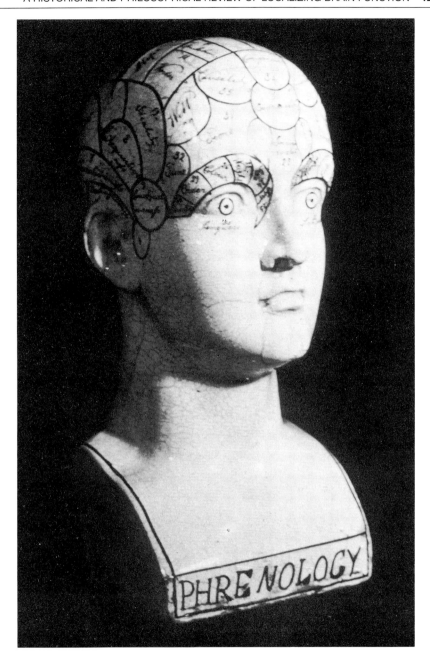

Fig 1. Phrenological view of localizing brain function. (From the collection of Dr. Michael Trimble)

discovering the location of the lesion that caused their symptom. However, the study of the dysfunction that occurs with ablative lesions in critical points of the brain only indirectly informs us about actual brain function. The study of dysfunction arising from strokes and tumours can only tell us which brain regions are absolutely critical for a specific behaviour. If a behaviour ceases with a certain lesion (for example, not being able to move your right arm after a lesion in the left motor strip), then that brain region is *necessary* for the behaviour, but it is not *sufficient* to produce it. Most brain regions act in concert with other regions to produce behaviour (see Chap. 6).

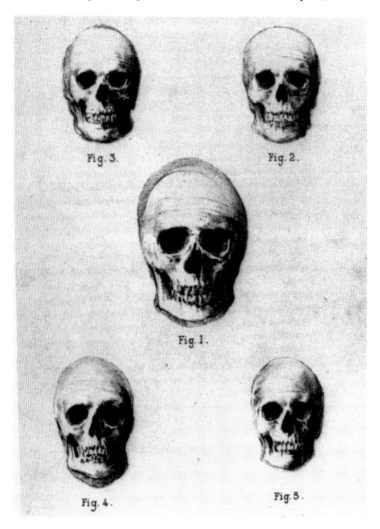

**Fig 2.** An early attempt at using 'neuroimaging' to diagnose pathology. At the beginning of the nineteenth century, the new technology of photography was used to try and identify the facial characteristics of criminals. Skull X-rays were taken from 12 criminals and overlaid, thus giving a composite of the 'criminal face'. (Photograph reproduced courtesy of Daniel Pick, Cambridge University Press.)

The same is true of the human cortical stimulation experiments carried out by Wilder Penfield (Penfield and Rasmussen 1950; Penfield and Jasper 1954). During neurosurgery, Penfield electrically stimulated various regions of the cortex and observed what happened in his awake patients. He was thus able to map the human cortex or map the products of electrical stimulation of the cortex. In a way this was one step closer to understanding true brain function than studying ablative lesions such as strokes and tumours. However, even these pioneering experiments did not reveal how the brain functioned in a coordinated way to produce different behaviours.

The discovery and development of the electroencephalogram in the early 1900s generated a great deal of anticipation about the possibility of better lesion and function localization. Unfortunately, the EEG has not lived up to these initial expectations, even with the recent advance of colour EEG mapping (BEAM). Although EEGs can localize specific seizure foci, the typical EEG does not change enough during most behaviours to attempt localization.

Before the advent of CT in the mid-1970s and MRI in the mid-1980s, the field of neuropsychology had a long tradition of locating destructive brain lesions based on patient performance on complex neuropsychological tests (Damasio and Damasio 1989). With the increased sensitivity of the powerful imaging techniques of CT and MRI, modern neuropsychology has largely abandoned its localization role. Interestingly, though, several investigators have recently breathed new life into this field by introducing complicated algorithms which produce a cortical map based on performance on neuropsychological tests (Gur et al. 1988; Yeo et al. 1990). A brain grid or map has been developed based on test score performance. Thus, if a patient performed poorly on a spatial task, the right parietal lobe 'activity' on the grid would be low.

The impact of these new neuropsychological algorithms on localizing brain function remains to be seen. Unquestionably, however, the field of clinical neuropsychology has advanced our knowledge of regional brain functions. These new computer-generated neuropsychological maps may continue this contribution.

Much of the work of understanding brain function remains ahead and is being done now with PET and SPET. However, combining the knowledge gained from destructive lesions, cortical stimulation, previous neuropsychological work, and early functional neuroimaging gives a rough estimate of some critical areas of the brain involved in certain behaviours. An outline version of this classic view is presented in Table 1.

## Philosophical Review

A working knowledge of the various theories concerning the interaction between the mind and brain can help to clarify thinking in the field of functional neuroimaging. Here we briefly examine different theories of mind-brain interaction. Originally, it was philosophers more than physicians who were occupied with theories of how the mind and brain work. In order to understand some of the present theories about the brain and the mind better, it is helpful to review the teachings of one of the most famous philosophers of all time, René Descartes (Descartes 1967).

**Table 1.** Brain function by location

| Brain region and (function) | Results of ablative lesion | Results of stimulation |
|---|---|---|
| *Frontal lobes* | Paralysis of contralateral face, arm and leg | Contraction of contralateral corresponding muscles |
| (Executive) | Pseudobulbar palsy, urinary and faecal incontinence | |
| (Planning, thinking) | Lack of spontaneity (abulia, akinetic mutism) | |
| | Coarsening of personality | |
| Broca's area | Agraphia, apraxia, motor speech disorder | |
| *Temporal lobes* | Visual field defect (contralateral upper homonymous quandrantanopia) | Olfactory sensations, emotional memories, Auditory hallucinations, |
| | Auditory deafness | Autonomic arousal, sexual aberrations |
| Dominant (left) | Wernicke's aphasia | |
| (Language) | Amusia | |
| Non-dominant (right) | Poor spatial relationships | |
| (Spatial, music) | Poor memory (Korsakoff's amnesic defect) | |
| | Kluver-Bucy syndrome (apathy, sham rage, increased sexual activity) | |
| *Parietal lobes* – (either) (Coordinating brain activity) | Contralateral hemianaesthesia Contralateral hemiparesis (mild) Visual field defect (homonymous hemianopia) | |
| (Dominant) | Alexia, apraxia, Gerstmann syndrome | |

Descartes tackled tough philosophical questions. He sought to know how we came to be (cosmological search) and how we come to know the world around us (epistemological search). He therefore sought to return to the basics or first principles and then prove how our minds and brains function. He did this with his famous dictum, *"Cogito ergo sum"* (I think therefore I am) (Descartes 1967). By examining his own thoughts (introspecting) and doubting everything, he finally arrived at a thought that he knew was true and undoubtable – namely that he was a thinking mind.

Now, how does this relate to functional neuroimaging? Because Descartes 'withdrew' philosophically into his mind, he forever felt that his mind was somehow dramatically different from his brain. Descartes argued that the mind – our thoughts, wishes, perceptions and desires – is somehow of a different nature than the body and the brain. The mind exists in a different or dual realm from the body and the two are hardly related (known as *Cartesian dualism*). Brain has extension in space whereas the mind does not. However, Descartes realized that somehow the mind must interact with the brain. He thought this connection between mind and brain occurs at the pineal gland, an organ Descartes believed existed only in man.

Thus, if Descartes had been given access to a high-resolution SPET scanner and had then been asked to predict what part of the brain was involved in making one's arm move, he would have likely predicted that the pineal gland would have demonstrated increased rCBF. Because of his underlying beliefs about how the mind interacts with the brain, he would have asked very different questions about the brain than we now do. One's underlying theory of mind-brain function determines the hypotheses that one tests. This point is important to remember in the realm of functional neuroimaging.

Although most modern neuroscientists dismiss Descartes' mind-brain dualism as a historical diversion, Descartes' influence remains powerful even today (Symthies and Beloff 1989). Only within the past century have many people believed something other than Cartesian dualism when thinking about the mind and its interaction with the brain (Ryle 1949) (see Table 2). Some view the Cartesian mind-brain split as one of the driving forces behind the separate development of the fields of neurology and psychiatry. Neurology as a specialty has largely dealt with the brain and its dysfunctions (a mindless brain), while psychiatry has until just recently occupied itself with the mind, divorced from the brain (a brainless mind). Recently, with the emergence of new technologies like SPET neuroimaging, the classic mind/brain, neurology/psychiatry distinctions are being rethought. But if one is not a Cartesian dualist believing that the mind and brain are separate, interacting perhaps through the pineal gland, what other ways are there for understanding how the mind (thoughts) and the brain interact?

Table 2. Different theories of mind-brain interaction

| Theory | Belief |
|---|---|
| Cartesian dualism | The mind and thoughts are separate from the brain and are of a different nature. The brain is physical, whereas thoughts are not. The two interact at the pineal gland, according to Descartes. |
| Behaviourism | One should not speak of the mind or attempt to understand the brain. One should only study observable behaviour. |
| Reductive materialism | With enough knowledge thoughts will someday be totally understood in terms of the human brain and interactions between neurons. We will be able to rethink and reforge psychology in terms of a powerful neuroscience. |
| Functionalism | Thoughts emerge from complex organization and are not necessarily specific to human neurons. Thus, computers or other life-forms could have thoughts and feelings. |

In the mid-1900s many people were philosophical and psychological *behaviourists* (Churchland 1988). In part because the brain was largely inaccessible, behaviourists understood the 'mind' strictly in terms of observable behaviour, that is, any statement about a mental state or thought could be better understood in terms of observable behaviour that would result from having such a thought or mental state. The mind was understood only in terms of behaviour and the brain was a 'black box' out of which behaviour mysteriously emerged. Although many of the principles of behaviourism remain, fortunately we can now open up the 'black box' of the brain with tools such as functional neuroimaging with SPET.

A commonly held modern view, and perhaps the 'opposite' of Cartesian dualism, is the theory of *reductive materialism* (Young 1986). A reductive materialist would argue that the mind or mental states can be reduced to physical states. That is, if we only knew enough, each thought or word or action could be totally understood in terms of the interactions of neurons in our brain. Accordingly, there is nothing about the mind that could not be explained if only we knew enough about the physical functioning of the brain. Our present psychological theories will be modified and expanded to someday explain the complex steps from genetic expression and neurochemistry to 'thoughts', 'beliefs' and behaviour. Many modern neuroscientists, if pushed, would probably call themselves reductive materialists. A reductive materialist view is the background for most neuroSPET and neuroPET research. In Chap. 6 we discuss several different modern theories about brain organization. This entire field gets somewhat more complicated, or interesting, depending on one's perspective, if one asks whether thoughts or the mind can come from the brain only, that is, are thoughts, feelings and emotions unique to organized neurons or could they also arise from other types of organization? Are there more ways than one for nature, and perhaps even man, to put together a thinking creature? A strict reductive materialist would argue that thoughts and feelings are somehow unique to organized neurons and that a complex computer could never have thoughts or a mind. Those who believe that thoughts and minds can emerge from complex structures other than neurons are *functionalists*, that is, thoughts and feelings are a function of complex organization and are not necessarily tied exclusively to human neurons. Thoughts are not understood strictly in terms of neurons, but instead, in terms of functional states that might correspond to neurons, or computer circuits, or whatever else might be able to 'think'. Thus, an extremely complex computer could have thoughts and feelings. Or, a life-form from another planet, non-carbon-based, and not having neurons, could theoretically have thoughts and a mind. Functionalists argue that thoughts emerge from complex organization and are not necessarily restricted to human neurons.

## Conclusion

Reviewing the history of man's attempts to localize brain function gives an appreciation of the power of functional neuroimaging to answer the questions that men have asked through the millennia. Additionally, one can see how functional neuroimaging may finally put an end to dualistic concepts, and the damage they have caused to neuroscientific progress. Functional neuroimaging constantly reminds us of the inextricable interactions and links between the mind and brain. In the next chapter we examine different theories of how the brain is organized and how that organization can be probed with functional neuroimaging.

# References

Churchland PS (1988) Neurophilosophy: toward a unified science of the mind-brain. The MIT Press, London
Damasio H, Damasio AR (1989) Lesion analysis in neuropsychology. Oxford University Press, New York
Descartes R (1967) Meditation, II. In: Haldane ES, Ross GRT (trans) The philosophical works of Descartes. Cambridge University Press, Cambridge
Gur RC, Trivedi SS, Saykin AJ, et al (1988) Behavioral imaging: a procedure for the analysis and display of neuropsychological test scores I. Construction of the algorithm and initial clinical evaluation. Neuropsychia, Neuropsychol Behav Neural 1:53–60
Hill EG, George MS (1987) The 'therapeutik method of headach' in the seventeenth century. Neurology 36:219(abstract)
Penfield W, Jasper H (1954) Epilepsy and the functional anatomy of the human brain. Little, Brown and Co., Boston
Penfield W, Rasmussen T (1950) The cerebral cortex of man. Macmillan, New York
Pick, D (1990) Faces of degeneration. Cambridge University Press, Cambridge
Ryle G (1949) The concept of mind. Hutchinson, London
Smythies JR, Beloff J (1989) The case for dualism. University Press of Virginia, Charlottesville, Virginia
Taylor J (1958) Selected writings of John Hughlings Jackson. Basic Books, New York
Trimble MR (1988) Biological psychiatry. John Wiley, Chichester
Yeo RA, Turkheimer E, Bigler ED (1990) Neuropsychological methods of localizing brain dysfunction: clinical versus empirical approaches. Neuropsychia, Neuropsychol Behav Neural 3:290–303
Young JZ (1986) Philosophy and the brain. Oxford University Press, Oxford

Chapter 6

# Models of Brain Processing with Respect to Functional Neuroimaging

## Introduction

The cerebral cortex contains approximately $10^{14}$ synapses (von der Malsburg and Singer 1988). Current neuroimaging techniques can only resolve brain regions containing millions of cells. Hence it is always the coordinated functioning of millions of synapses and neurons that generate measurable activity. A single neuron cannot alone accomplish the processing from which complex behaviours emerge. Thus, in attempting to understand the neuronal basis of complex behaviour it is essential to have a theoretical model of the interactions of large groups of functional units. This not only makes data management convenient; it also in some way represents biological reality.

In the investigation of patterns of regional cerebral blood flow in the diseased brain scanned in a single state, a purely descriptive account of the findings may provide adequate information about the disease in question. For example, the simple delineation of a region of decreased blood flow in a patient with focal epilepsy scanned interictally may fulfil the requirements of the scan. However, if the aim of the study is to provide understanding of the dynamic processes underlying complex behaviours, then both the study protocol and the subsequent data analysis will require a different structure. In the first place, if the basis of a particular behaviour is to be investigated, then it is not sufficient to scan the subject only during the performance of that behaviour. This is because the scan will be a measure of the subject's total cerebral activity at the time of scanning. Thus, the behaviour of interest will not be the only act that the individual is engaging in during the scan. There will be both related and unrelated activities coexisting with the target activity. Hence if the required behaviour is listening to spoken words, the ongoing functional state of the brain will be maintaining the individual in an awake and alert state, generating selective attention and directing it to the task in hand, suppressing alternative activities, thinking generally about the nature of the task, perhaps suffering anxiety at the stress or discomfort of participating in the study, considering the meaning of the words being presented and probably many other things as well. Thus, in order to isolate the changes in cerebral activity specifically associated with the behaviour of interest, it is necessary to scan the subject in a control state that will seek to be identical to the test state apart from this one activity. If it is desired to isolate different components of a complex task, then a number of different control or comparison states will require investigation, either within the same protocol or across a number of studies, each comparing only two conditions.

Analysis of the results of such an investigation will involve the comparison of at least two data sets, each describing activity in a different state. The results of such a comparison may be that one or more parts of the brain demonstrate either increased or decreased activity associated with the change in state. However, in order to be able to attribute meaning to these results it is necessary to apply some theoretical model of brain function to them. This is of particular importance if activity is found to change in more than one area. If this is the case, then a number of questions must immediately be asked. Firstly, are all the regional changes in activity associated with task performance or do some of them reflect artefacts of the investigation, such as alteration in subject positioning between the scans or an inadequatae control task that fails to match all but the index task? Secondly, if more than one region is involved then how do we interpret the association between these regions? Is it sufficient simply to record the variations in all these regions or should the nature of the relationship between these sites of changing activity be investigated using a correlational analysis? Thirdly, if brain regions are correlated in their activity and we fail to appreciate this, then how may this error affect the conclusions drawn from the study? Refinement and careful analysis of the study protocol may help to answer the first issue but the second and third questions require the application of some model of brain functioning within which to interpret the results. Considering the most simple example of repeated 'resting' scans in the same subjects carried out with xenon 133 (Prohovnik et al. 1980), correlations were found between the blood-flow rates of contralateral homologous brain regions. In a positron emission tomography (PET) study of normal volunteers, Mettler et al. (1984) examined correlations within 26 brain regions during resting fluorine-18 fluorodeoxyglucose scans. Using a correlation matrix for the 26 regions of interest, two apparently separate functional systems were identified. The dangers of neglecting or failing to recognize interhemispheric regional correlations has been considered by Clark et al. (1985) from the perspective of searching for evidence of cerebral asymmetries of function. These authors point out that the probability of finding evidence to support a cerebral specialization model of brain function is dependent, in part, on the degree of cerebral integration when within-subject comparisons are performed. This is the case because as the degree of cross-hemisphere integration increases, the left-to-right comparisons show a smaller difference. As this correlation approaches unity, progressively smaller differences between left and right hemisphere activities will become significant. Hence an apparent asymmetry of function may in reality be a function of strong interhemispheric integration.

The two statistical approaches – the search for discrete regions of changed activity, or for patterns of correlations between regions – are not mutually exclusive and the methods utilized should depend on the nature of the function being investigated and the model of brain processing that is employed. For more complex tasks correlational analyses are more likely to contribute important information about the neural basis of performance.

However, even this simple statement makes an assumption about brain functioning: specifically that there are functionally discrete brain regions that may or may not act in concert, depending on the task in hand.

It is now appropriate to consider briefly models of brain function that may be either implicit or explicit in the interpretation of changes in cerebral activity associated with the performance of complex behaviours (Table 1). It has been pointed out (Lashley 1937) that, because of the enormous complexity of the brain, descriptions of its function have tended to be formulated in terms of the most sophisticated technology of the day: from ideas of aqueduct-like flows of bodily humours in ancient Greece and Rome, through Sherrington's analogy of a telephone switchboard, to modern concepts based on computer models of artificial intelligence. The related factors of both location and nature of cerebral processes have been subjects of a sustained debate, the history of which is reviewed in Chap. 5. With respect to recent views of the localization of brain functions, two opposing views may be summarized. Lashley (1937), while accepting that for cyto-architectural or neurophysiological reasons there were discrete brain regions with particular functions, was of the opinion that "conceptions of the organization of the mind or of behaviour are based on a logical analysis of the activities of the total organism, and the final synthesis of nervous states which constitute these activities must transcend the excitation of any single centre". He concluded that a particular behavioural disturbance could not be ascribed to a brain region, that the degree to which skilled movement is impaired is directly related to the mass of brain damaged, and that different areas of the cerebral cortex are equipotential with respect to complex functions. Geschwind (1965 a,b), on the other hand, particularly in his analysis of language disorders, emphasized the roles of specific brain regions with particular functions (the primary receptive and motor speech areas) and the importance of the anatomical connections between these regions. This approach emphasized the observation that if more than one brain region is involved in the generation of a behaviour, then the nature of the interaction between the areas must also be understood.

Table 1. Models of complex brain functioning

| Model | Central features |
|---|---|
| A. Location of activity | |
| Lashley – mass action | Activity in volumes of brain |
| | Cortex is equipotential for complex functions |
| Geschwind – connectionism | The interaction of functionally discrete brain systems and their connections |
| B. Nature of processing | |
| Serial | The high speed repetition of essentially simple operations |
| | Increased or ambiguous constraints slow processing |
| Parallel | Simultaneous consideration of many items in different sites |
| | Constraints may aid processing |
| | Solutions are an emergent property of the system |

# The Parallel Distributed Processing Model of Brain Function

When considering the nature of complex cerebral processing, current ideas have progressed from the assembly-line model of Descartes, which involved the serial processing of information along a hierarchy of dedicated centres. Now theories of parallel distributed processing (PDP) based in interconnected neural networks (Mesulam 1990) are generating increasing interest.

It is understandable that brain function is expressed in the high technology of the day, but this expectation should not devalue the current ideas. Theories of PDP appear to have sufficient face validity to warrant further exploration. Additionally, they have implications for hypothesis generation and image interpretation in functional neuroimaging.

The phrase "parallel distributed processing" was coined by McClelland, Rumelhart and colleagues and it sought to emphasize not only the parallel nature of the processing, but also the use of distributed representation and distributed control of processes. Single cyto-architectonic fields or immediately contiguous areas form the local neural networks that are the building-blocks of larger systems for the PDP of complex behaviours (Mesulam 1990). Such networks have been described subserving, for example, the analysis of shape and spatial location (Lehky and Sejnowski 1988; Zipser and Andersen 1988).

The properties of networks have been thoroughly discussed by a number of authors (Rumelhart et al. 1986; Churchland 1989; Crick 1989). A theoretical neural network is displayed in Fig. 1. In this very simple model there are only three levels: an input or sensory layer, a middle layer composed of 'hidden units' and an output layer. Each unit in the first two layers connects to all units

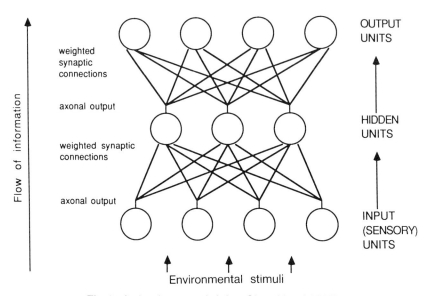

Fig 1. A simple network (after Churchland 1989).

in the layer above. In this very basic model there are no reverse or sideways connections. The input units, analogous to sensory neurons, each receive a particular state of activation from an environmental stimulus. The activity in each unit represents a particular aspect of the environment, and the activation level across all the input units forms the whole representation of the input situation at that time. The input activation levels are then propagated upwards to the hidden units. Each such unit sums the inputs reaching it and the resultant activity is then propagated to the output units. The organization of the network allows it to learn how to analyse various inputs in such a way as to come to the correct conclusions. The learning process is brought about by the application of a theoretical rule that generates learning by the back-propagation of error (Rumelhart et al. 1986). This involves the repeated modulation of initially random synaptic weights of the connections between the units of different layers by indicating to each unit the size and sign of its error in repeated performances of the task and the required correction. By this means the repeated small adjustments in the strength of each synapse gradually reduce the total error in the performance of the whole net (Crick 1989).

The attraction of this model is that the application of a simple rule to a simple network of interconnected units allows complex learning. The limitations of the model are that there is as yet no known brain mechanism to calculate the partial corrections required to train the system and no clear means by which these correction messages are passed back down the network to the relevant synaptic connections. In experimental models the 'teaching' is performed by an external computer. However, as discussed by Churchland (1989), there is an alternative model which may explain learning in biological networks of neurons. Hebb described the mechanism found in brains by which the weight of a synaptic connection is increased in the presence of a temporal coincidence, on either side of a given synaptic junction, of a strong signal in the afferent axon and a high level of excitation in the receiving cell, that is, the synapse is strengthened if it receives an input signal on the pre-synaptic side and some activity, such as unit firing, on the post-synaptic side. It has been demonstrated that such a system may lead to learning in an artificial network of orientation-selection cells (Linsker 1986). The advantage of this model is that there is no need for the calculation and back-propagation of errors.

While the activity within a local network is likely to be below the limits of detection by current neuroimaging techniques, the activity of multifocal neuronal systems composed of interconnected neural networks may be measurable. Complex tasks require the consideration and processing of a number of constituent elements. According to models of PDP the analysis of these elements is mapped onto multiple processors. While the factors determining the precise pattern of mapping are complex (Nelson and Bower 1990), large-scale networks subserving complex cognitive functions such as directed attention, language and memory have been proposed (Mesulam 1990; Nelson and Bower 1990). These systems operate by rules formulated in work by Rumelhart et al. (1986). Parallel processing describes a mode of computation in which many constraints and items of information are considered simultaneously by numbers of relatively simple processing units that are highly interconnected and that operate in parallel. Problems are solved by iteratively seeking to satisfy a number of constraints, so that the system can relax into a state of least conflict. Within each network weak constraints represent small synaptic weights and stronger constraints larger weights. By this means the processing of a problem accelerates as additional constraints become exploited. Each constraint may be imperfectly specified and ambiguous, yet each may play a potentially decisive role in determining the outcome of the process. In this way each aspect of the information describing a situation can act on other aspects, simultaneously influencing and being influenced by them. Such a property shows closer resemblance to recognized brain functioning than do models of serial processing in which processing slows down as the number of constraints increases. A problem may be solved without an overview of its nature but just by a number of simple processors, each attempting to honour the constraints set upon it. The resultant solution is not the sequential sum of each process but rather an emergent quality of the system as a whole.

There are, however, temporal limits to parallel processing. When an input enters the system, the system relaxes to accommodate it, that is, a representation is made of the input during which the input is processed. However, when a new input arrives, the state of the system will change again. Rumelhart and colleagues suggest that the relaxation procedure, together with the time spent in the resulting stable state, occupies about half a second. They conclude that events requiring less than half a second are processed in a purely parallel manner, while those taking longer involve a series of such processes and therefore have a serial component. Hence a brief complex behaviour such as the semantic analysis of a single word may be accomplished entirely by parallel processing. However, the production of a sentence of speech requires the temporal development of a series of processes, together with an ongoing appreciation of the state of that development.

Applying these concepts to the human brain has a number of implications. PDP theories assume that a complex behaviour is represented in multiple sites and that each site is likely to have a role in many different behaviours. Hence lesions in different parts of the brain may lead to disturbances of various aspects of the same overall behaviour while a single lesion may result in deficits in multiple behaviours. An example taken from models described by Mesulam (1990) may serve to clarify these ideas. Destructive cerebral lesions such as tumours and cerebrovascular accidents may lead to a syndrome of inability to direct attention towards motivationally relevant segments of extrapersonal space. Mesulam utilized this class of disorder to explore an extended network for the distribution of directed attention. On the basis of clinical and experimental studies, he concluded that cortical lesions consistently leading to neglect have been described in three areas: the dorsolateral posterior parietal cortex, the dorsolateral premotor prefrontal cortex and the cingulate gyrus. It is noted that these areas are linked to each other by extensive and reciprocal monosynaptic connections. There are additional subcortical regions where lesions may cause neglect that are connected to at least two of these three cortical foci. Mesulam suggests that directed attention is organized in a distributed large-scale network across these regions, with each region contributing a different aspect to the processing of the environment. The parietal component generates a sensory representation, the frontal cortex a map for orienting and exploration and the cingulate introduces a set of values into the regions of close extrapersonal space. Animal studies support the notion that specific lesions in one of these areas disturb directed spatial attention in the predicted manner. These regions are arranged in what is described as a 'dyadic hub and spoke' network in which the three cortical sites are interconnected directly and via two subcortical sites. The processing of extrapersonal space may thus be thought of as existing in three planes distributed across these sites (Fig. 2). The first plane is the anatomical structure supporting the processing. It consists of local neural nets in the sites defined above. The second plane represents the neural processing within these sites. This processing is parallel in that it occurs simultaneously in each site, and it is distributed in space within the brain. The interconnections between the local nets in the first plane mean that the processes in the second plane are no longer independent of one another. The third and final plane, representing the animal behaviour resulting from the activity in the first two planes, illustrates that although directed attention is composed of a number of elements, the nature of the behaviour is a result of the interactions between the component sites. Mesulam interprets these observations as suggesting that the anatomical mapping of behaviour is both localized and distributed but neither equipotential nor modular.

This model of brain activity explains why neuroimaging of complex behaviours is likely to detect multiple areas of activation in association with individual complex behaviours. This is important when imaging behaviours in normal volunteers, but it becomes even more so when examining the effects of pathological states on task performance. In pathological states it may not be predictable, from the site of the lesion, how regional cerebral activities will change during task performance. Preconceived notions regarding the pattern of activation may result in failure to recognize significant alterations in this pattern. On the other hand, the absence of an a priori hypothesis means that analysis of the results will involve multiple tests of significance to reveal regions of changed activity. In this case it will be necessary to employ the appropriate statistical corrections or use a sufficiently high threshold of significance.

Two examples drawn from recent neuroimaging studies of complex cognition may help to demonstrate the value of an appropriate model of brain functioning in interpreting findings. Roland and Friberg (1985) investigated the localization of cortical areas activated by thinking, having constructed an operational definition of thinking as "brain work in the form of operations on internal information, done by an awake subject". Arithmetic, auditory and visual memory tasks were investigated using intracarotid $^{133}$Xe injection and the measurement of regional cerebral blood flow (rCBF) in 254 cortical regions. In each task multiple cortical fields were activated. The authors concluded that since the three types of thinking produced different patterns of activation, the forms of thinking were different. They also noted that these results did not conform to a serial transmission model of information flow. However, in the absence of a theoretical model by which to interpret the finding of multiple sites of activation, although it was possible to describe changes in brain activity associated with the tasks, the authors did not dissect out the shared and different features of the tasks which may have contributed to a greater understanding of the processes involved in 'thinking'. In a PET study (measuring rCBF after bolus injections of oxygen-15 $H_2O$) of the cortical anatomy of single word processing, Petersen et al. (1988) investigated the effects of visual and auditory presentation, repetition and the semantic

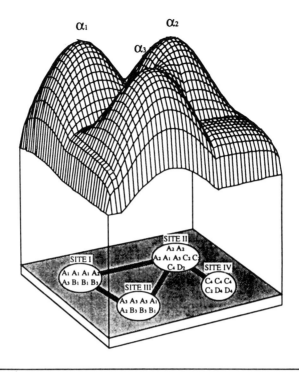

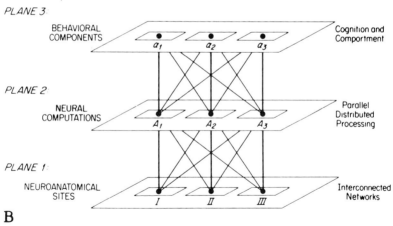

processing of words. Each task resulted in the activation of a different set of regions. In this way the results are analogous to those of Roland and Friberg described above. However, while the latter authors limited themselves to describing the different patterns of cerebral activity associated with the different tasks, Petersen and colleagues applied the concept of parallel processing to derive a distributed network subserving different forms of lexical processing. While such a network remains far from proven, it represents an attempt to use neuroimaging to understand the mechanisms of cognition rather than just the anatomical location of various cerebral processes.

# Conclusions

If functional neuroimaging is to be used as a tool in the analysis of complex behaviours, then simply describing which parts of the brain appear to be involved in these processes will not enhance our understanding of the underlying mechanisms of these behaviours. In order to attribute meaning to the observed results it is necesary to apply some conception of how the brain copes with complex tasks. The models utilized come in the first instance from clinical and experimental observations of the behavioural consequences of brain damage. These models may then be used to generate hypotheses which can be tested using functional neuroimaging. Ultimately, functional neuroimaging may be able to develop these hypotheses further, but to begin with we must be able to make sense of the intriguing and complex images provided by this technology. Parallel distributed processing is currently the most versatile and life-like model of brain information processing. It may lead to greater understanding of the cerebral nature of complex behaviours, but at the moment it should be remembered that it is still only a model.

**Fig 2 (*opposite*). A** The schematic relationships between anatomical site, neural computation, and behaviour. Sites I, II, and III collectively constitute a large-scale network underlying behaviour $\alpha$. Thus, $\alpha1$, $\alpha2$, and $\alpha3$ components define the behavioural plane. Site I is most closely associated with $\alpha1$, Site II with $\alpha2$, and Site III with $\alpha3$, but the relationship is not one to one and contains considerable eccentricity. **B** The vertical relationship between the neuroanatomical, computational, and behavioural planes. *Thick lines* indicate strong interactions, and *lighter lines* indicate weaker interactions. This configuration reconciles reductionism with emergence; reductionism represents a top-down perspective from behaviour to computation and to neuron structure, whereas emergence results from looking at the same interactions from a bottom-up perspective. The additional features that emerge during the upward ascent from one level to the next represent the relational architecture among the components and cannot be reduced to a simple list of lower-level constituents. Reproduced, with permission, from Mesulam (1990).

# References

Churchland PM (1989) A neurocomputational perspective. MIT Press, Cambridge, Massachusetts, pp 153–230

Clark CM, Kessler R, Margolin R (1985) The statistical interaction of cerebral specialization and integration in the interpretation of dynamic brain images. Brain Cogn 4:7–12

Crick F (1989) The recent excitement about neural networks. Nature 337:129–132

Geschwind N (1965a) Disconnexion syndromes in animals and man. Brain 88:237–294

Geschwind N (1965b) Disconnexion syndromes in animals and man. Brain 88:585–644

Lashley KS (1937) Functional determinants of cerebral localization. Arch Neurol Psychiatry 38:371–387

Lehky SR, Sejnowski TR (1988) Network model of shape-from-shading: neural function arises from both receptive and projective fields. Nature 333:452–454

Linsker R (1986) From basic network principles to neural architecture: emergence of orientation columns. Proc Natl Acad Sci 83:8779–8783

Malsburg C von der, Singer W (1988) Principles of cortical network organization. In: Rakic P, Singer W (eds) Neurobiology of neocortex. John Wiley, Chichester, pp 69–99

Mesulam M-M (1990) Large-scale neurocognitive networks and distributed processing for attention, language and memory. Ann Neurol 28:597–613

Mettler EJ, Riege WH, Kuhl DE (1984) Cerebral metabolic relationships for selected brain regions in healthy adults. J Cereb Blood Flow Metab 4:1–7

Nelson ME, Bower JM (1990) Brain maps and parallel computers. Trends Neurosci 13:403–408

Petersen SE, Fox PT, Posner MI (1988) Positron emission tomographic studies of the cortical anatomy of single-word processing. Nature 331:585–589

Prohovnik I, Hakansson K, Risberg J (1980) Observations on the functional significance of regional cerebral blood flow in "resting" normal subjects. Neuropsychologia 18:203–217

Roland PE, Friberg L (1985) Localization of cortical areas activated by thinking. J Neurophysiol 53:1219–1243

Rumelhart DE, McClelland JL, The PDP research group (1986) Parallel distributed processing, vol 1. MIT Press, Cambridge

Zipser D, Andersen RA (1988) A back-propagation programmed network that simulates response properties of a sub-set of posterior parietal neurones. Nature 331:676–684

Chapter 7
# Description and Principles of Neuroactivation

## Introduction

Recent advances in our knowledge of the local patterns of brain functional activity began with the studies of Lassen (Lassen et al. 1978) who developed techniques to measure blood flow in circumscribed regions of the intact human brain with the aid of radioactive isotopes. Even in the early studies, which required carotid artery cannulation and which had poor resolution by modern standards, Lassen and his colleagues demonstrated specific repeatable patterns of cortical blood flow associated with particular states and tasks. More recently the development of positron emission tomography (PET) and single-photon emission tomography (SPET) has further revolutionized our ability to view the living, working human brain.

Much of the work up to the present time has been concerned with visualizing brain function with the subject in a single state, often at rest. However, it is also possible to image the brain before and after the performance of particular tasks. The aim of such studies is to identify regional alterations in brain activity that are associated with performance of the task in question. By this means the cerebral bases of these tasks may be investigated. This approach is of value in both health and disease. In normal volunteers it is possible to investigate regional and neurophysiological responses to pharmacological or behavioural stimuli (see Chaps. 8 and 9). In patients it is possible to investigate the effects of pathological states on cerebral processes (see Chap. 10). The results of patient studies have clinical utility, as a way of defining the extent and nature of the disease process, and potentially they also have academic interest since the effects of known pathologies on cerebral processes may shed light on the mechanisms of these processes, much as post-traumatic brain lesion studies have helped in the understanding of normal brain function. Although not currently exploited to any great extent, it is also possible that an activation protocol may help in the diagnosis of a disease state by its use as a form of 'stress test' to exaggerate more subtle pathological changes. Thus, it is not surprising that activation techniques have been described as among the most interesting potential applications of blood flow studies (Andreasen 1988). But despite their great utility they are fraught with methodological difficulties, and a review of the published activation studies using SPET demonstrates many problems and differences in practice.

Once it is established for a specific imaging technique that a task detectably and consistently activates particular brain regions in normals, one can then examine the cerebral response patterns to such a stimulus in patients with psychiatric and neurological disease (Mazziotta and Phelps 1984). For instance, using a xenon-133 inhalation technique with multiple head probes to measure regional cortical blood flow, Weinberger et al. (1986) demonstrated that patients with chronic schizophrenia failed to increase blood flow to dorsolateral prefrontal cortex during performance of the Wisconsin Card Sort test while this change was observed in normal controls. Although some PET activation studies have used other indices of cerebral activity, for instance changes in glucose metabolic rate (Mazziotta and Phelps 1986), most SPET studies have concentrated on measures of blood flow.

## Methodological Issues

In essence, an activation study requires the comparison of at least two data sets describing brain activity generated in conditions that differ for the specific function in question. In designing an activation protocol a number of decisions must be made. These include the nature of the activation regime, the tracer ligand to be utilized, the SPET instrument and the method of subsequent data analysis. Variations in any of these will greatly affect the results.

### Activation Procedures

The choice of activation and control conditions depends on the question being asked but this choice is also constrained by the technical requirements of the methods to be used.

In terms of the question to be answered, some studies (Biersack et al. 1987; Matsuda et al. 1988; Battisstin et al. 1989; Dahl et al. 1989) have been directly concerned with the effect on regional cerebral blood flow of a particular stimulus. Others (Goldenberg et al. 1987, 1989; Lang et al. 1988; Walker-Batson et al. 1988) have observed the changes in cerebral blood flow associated with a stimulus to infer aspects of cerebral function that underlie the response to the stimulus. Activation techniques that have been used in SPET studies may be divided into three modalities: sensorimotor, cognitive and pharmacological. But regardless of the type of study, all activation tasks must share several qualities. They must generate a detectable and reproducible change in cerebral blood flow and ideal tasks must be controlled, sustainable and repeatable. It is not always obvious which tasks will best produce these changes. Ginsberg et al. (1987) used PET to measure the effects of a range of somatosensory stimuli on local glucose utilization rates. They found that the greatest activation resulted from tasks that required an active perceptual effort by the patient, while vigorous purely sensory stimulation failed to produce a consistent focus of activation. However, a recent account of activation of the human visual cortex by the observation of stroboscopic light reports that this protocol resulted in a local peak increase in radiopharmaceutical distribution of 36.7% (Woods et al. 1991). This large change in regional activity suggests that some passive sensory tasks can, in fact, produce significant activation. However, it should be noted that stroboscopic stimulation generates increased neuronal activity in a manner different to other passive sensory tasks. The phenomenon is made use of in routine electroencephalographic assessment of brain epileptiform activity.

## Motor Activation Studies

Purely motor activation tasks, for instance repeating voluntary movements, have not been well reported with SPET technology, although finger movements and learned motor tasks have been described in PET studies seeking to map cerebral representations of motor function (Mazziotta and Phelps 1986). Elsewhere in this book we describe the recent demonstration of human parietal cortex activation associated with a task involving fine finger movements.

## Pharmacological Activation Studies

Pharmacological activation studies may be used to learn about the cerebral actions of the administered drug. Alternatively, the known cerebral effects of a substance that requires or activates specific brain regions or functions may allow examination of these particular systems. Thus, an investigation into cholinergic involvement in the memory deficits of Alzheimer's dementia (Battisstin et al. 1989) utilized the cholinomimetic properties of L-acetylcarnitine to observe the effects of increasing cholinergic activity on regional, particularly parietal, cerebral blood flow in patients with this condition (see Chap. 10). Pharmacological techniques provide a new means for investigating cerebrovascular disease. A number of studies have examined the results of challenging the cerebral vasculature with substances that have vasodilating effects. Dahl et al. (1989) examined the response to nitroglycerin in dilating cerebral vasculature in part as an investigation into the therapeutic actions of this drug. Other substances having similar effects have also been utilized in activation paradigms. The inhalation of 7% carbon dioxide may produce side-effects such as nausea, tachycardia and increased blood pressure (Delecluse et al. 1989). Acetazolamide, on the other hand, is a powerful but harmless vasodilator that exerts its effects within 10 min following intravenous injection (Chollet et al. 1989; Delecluse et al. 1989), increasing regional cerebral blood flow in normal tissue by approximately 35% (Batjer et al. 1988). It has been used to study cerebral blood flow reactivity in patients with transient ischaemic attacks (TIAs) (Chollet et al. 1989), significantly increasing the sensitivity of SPET for detecting regions of pathological blood flow. The technique has also enabled the demonstration of hypoperfusion and impaired vasoreactivity in occipital and cerebellar regions in a patient with vertebrobasilar insufficiency (Delecluse et al. 1989).

As discussed below, the tracer kinetics in the techniques utilized mean that the task performance must be maintained for between 5 (Matsuda et al. 1988) and 20 min (Goldenberg et al. 1987). This is relatively straightforward for a procedure such as occlusion of a carotid artery (Matsuda et al. 1988), or for pure motor tasks, but it is more difficult for cognitive and abstract tasks such as thinking (Roland and Friberg 1985) or imagining faces (Goldenberg et al. 1989). The variability introduced by changes in the manner of performance of the study task between individuals may confound results and should ideally be both minimized and measured. It is also difficult to quantify exactly how much attention the subject devotes to performance of the task. Roland and Friberg (1985), in an intracarotid $^{133}$Xe injection study, attempted to tackle this problem by giving a task such as silent serial subtraction of 3's from 50 and then asking the subjects after a period of performance what answer they had reached. Goldenberg et al. (1989), after the completion of each of the test conditions questioned their subjects about the nature of mental activity during the tests. In one of the tasks described by Walker-Batson et al. (1988), however, requiring silent arithmetic calculation, there was no external measure of how well the subject was attending to the task.

## Choice of Control Task

In activation studies the relevant findings are the differences in regional cerebral blood flow between the test and the control tasks. The choice of control task is thus of critical importance. Since all aspects of physical and mental state may affect cerebral activity (Mazziotta and Phelps 1986), it is necessary that they be taken into account. Ideally, the only differences between the task and the control situation are those functions that are the focus of investigation. Many complex behaviours, for instance the use of language, are composed of multiple distinct but related processes. In such circumstances simply comparing speaking with not speaking will not isolate the separate tasks that contribute to the overall behaviour and which may be separately involved in various disease states. In order to circumvent this problem it is necessary to perform a number of different studies, each examining one aspect of the overall behaviour or, if possible, more than two conditions in the scan protocol. The latter solution is possible in PET studies that use radioisotopes with very short half-lives, for instance $^{15}$O with a half-life of 123 s (Petersen et al. 1988). However, the much longer half-life of $^{99m}$Tc (6 h) means that multiple doses cannot be given in the same protocol if sufficient radioactivity is administered to enable adequate data acquisition, even when prolonging the scan duration. In practice, with appropriate instrumentation, splitting the standard dose in half provides adequate signal and allows two studies to be performed without leading to a scan time so prolonged that it introduces other confounding factors, for example the increasing frustration or drowsiness of the subject by the time the next task is to be performed.

These observations emphasize the importance of validating activation paradigms on normal volunteers before drawing conclusions about the results of studies in groups with pathology. In addition, they demonstrate the difficulty of selecting a control situation that truly allows isolation of just the effects of the task or procedure in question.

## Choice of Tracer

Three different radioactive tracers have been used in published SPET neuroactivation studies: xenon-133, $^{123}$I-iodoamphetamine ($^{123}$IMP) and $^{99m}$Tc-D,L-hexamethylpropylene amine oxime (HMPAO). New tracers are currently being developed, several of which are aimed at particular neurotransmitter systems (see Chap. 2).

$^{99m}$Tc-HMPAO is a lipophilic substance that readily crosses the blood-brain barrier (Andersen et al. 1988). Its distribution following intravenous injection conforms closely to that of an ideal first-pass high-clearance marker of brain blood flow (Costa et al. 1986). Inside the brain it is rapidly converted to a hydrophilic form that is retained for many hours (Sharp et al. 1986). With respect to the use of $^{99m}$Tc-HMPAO as a blood-flow tracer for activation studies, important issues are the time course of its entrapment in the brain and its subsequent radioactive decay rate. These define the temporal relationships between tracer injection, task performance and image acquisition for each condition within the activation paradigm. In addition, the sensitivity of the detection apparatus and an acceptable upper limit to the total dose of administered radioactivity define the number of injections, and hence number of conditions, that may be given in the course of a study. In practice this is generally two: a control and an activation task.

It has been demonstrated using intracarotid injections of $^{99m}$Tc-HMPAO in human volunteers (Lassen et al. 1988) that total hemispheric counts reached a maximum within seconds then declined exponentially over 10 min to a steady-state representing 40-50% of peak activity. Hence investigators have used study designs in which the task is commenced 30 s (Matsuda et al. 1988) to 3 min (Lang et al. 1988) before intravenous injection of $^{99m}$Tc-HMPAO and continued for 4–7 min after injection. Image acquisition was then begun either immediately after cessation of task performance (Lang et al. 1988; Matsuda et al. 1988; Goldenberg et al. 1989) or after a delay of some minutes or hours when activation involved administration of an active drug (Biersack et al. 1987; Battisstin et al. 1989).

Andersen et al. (1988) have reported that once this steady-state is achieved, then further radioactivity is only lost slowly at a rate of 0.4% per hour. This observation has led to two designs of activation studies using $^{99m}$Tc-HMPAO. Some investigators performed the two conditions between 1 and 2 weeks apart, after cerebral radioactivity had returned to background levels (Biersack et al. 1987; Lang et al. 1988; Battisstin et al. 1989; Goldenberg et al. 1989). The potential to do this is important if the first condition performed involves the administration of a pharmacologically active substance with a significant duration of action. However, performing scans this far apart increases the likelihood that differences between the two scans are due to some factor unrelated to the activation procedure, for instance recent consumption of substances affecting cerebral blood flow such as caffeine or nicotine, or change in level of fatigue or affective state (Mazziotta and Phelps 1984; Lange et al. 1988) during the intervening period. In principle, the effects of these variables can be minimized by alternating the order of control and test tasks in different subjects within the study, as was done by Goldenberg et al. (1989) and Lang et al. (1988a).

To avoid the introduction of confounding variables arising from a prolonged interval between scans some investigators have performed both control and test scans within the same study session (Matsuda et al. 1988; also see Chap. 9). This method makes use of the observations described above that from 2 min after an injection of $^{99m}$Tc-HMPAO brain radioactivity levels remain more or less constant for several hours. Hence it is known after the first scan what the level of brain radioactivity is at the time of the second injection. The radioactivity of $^{99m}$Tc-HMPAO changes with time after preparation so that equal doses of radioactivity in the two injections do not guarantee equal doses of $^{99m}$Tc-HMPAO. Matsuda et al. (1988) resolved this problem by using ipsilateral cerebellar hemisphere activity as a reference value, noting that this was only valid because in this study cerebellar activity was itself unaffected by the activation procedure. Most reported $^{99m}$Tc-HMPAO studies have described blood flow indirectly. This is because quantitation of absolute blood flow values is difficult owing to early rapid movements of the tracer between blood and brain (Matsuda et al. 1988).

Xenon-133 inhalation has been used to measure cerebral blood flow in SPET activation protocols (Walker-Batson et al. 1988; Dahl et al. 1989). The advantages of this method are that there is less radiation exposure during the course of the study and that cerebral blood flow may be quantified in millilitres/gram per minute. With rapid washout, studies may be repeated after as little as 20 min. Walker-Batson et al. (1988) took advantage of these benefits to measure cerebral blood flow in four different tasks. Disadvantages of xenon activation include poorer resolution (16–20 mm full width at half maximum) (Andersen et al. 1988) and significant airway artefact, particularly when visualizing the cerebellum. Significant assumptions are made, such as fixed partition coefficients, for normal and diseased tissue.

$^{123}$I-IMP has also been used to measure cerebral blood flow during activation. However, following intravenous injection it takes about 20 min to reach steady-state. Distribution of $^{123}$I-IMP is then proportional to the regional cerebral blood flow during the time the steady-state was achieved (Goldenberg et al. 1987). Hence in an $^{123}$I-IMP activation protocol it is necessary to continue the activation and control tasks for at least 20 min. This not only limits suitable tasks but also introduces variables that are difficult to control such as fluctuations in task performance and overall state of arousal during the task.

In summary, $^{99m}$Tc-HMPAO appears to be the best commercially available tracer ligand for routine SPET activation procedures due to its rapid deposition in the active brain. Xenon-133, because of its poor image-resolution qualities, and $^{123}$I-IMP, because of its delayed brain uptake, are less preferable.

## Choice of SPET Instrument (see Chap. 3)

The recent development of brain-dedicated SPET instruments has increased the number and variety of neurophysiological tasks that may be performed with radiotracers available.

In summary, single detector systems are almost a technology of the past. Multiple-detector single-slice systems are useful for the initial study of new tracers and drugs. The new multiple-detector-head gamma cameras are ideal for neurophysiological activation tasks because of ease of patient positioning, multislice capability, and the improved sensitivity and efficiency of photon detection. Lower doses of radiotracers may be administered and subdivided, and scan acquisition times are shorter.

## Data Analysis

The majority of the SPET activation studies discussed here have measured the changing blood flow on activation in predetermined regions of interest (ROI) and then compared these ROI results during control and test conditions. In $^{99m}$Tc-HMPAO studies Goldenberg et al. (1989) and Lang et al. (1988a) used relative count rates obtained for each region of interest (ROI) by dividing the tracer concentration in that region by the mean count rate of all regions taken together. Matsuda et al. (1988) and Battistin et al. (1989) expressed activity as a ratio of activity in each ROI to the mean count rate over the cerebellum, corrected for early diffusion of tracer. Neither method is without drawbacks. The former dilutes the size of an activation effect in any specific region while the latter rests on the assumption that the cerebellum is itself not activated by the test procedure. The results were then discussed either purely as the size of change in flow in ROIs between conditions (Biersack et al. 1987; Walker-Batson et al. 1988), or examined for significance with $t$-tests (Lang et al. 1988; Battisstin et al. 1989). In a study with several activation tasks, comparisons between stimulated conditions across individuals were examined using analysis of variance techniques (Goldenberg et al. 1987).

These investigations of individual responses of discrete brain regions are based on the assumption that higher cognitive functions are performed by distinct brain regions working independently (Goldenberg et al. 1987). However, many argue that the bases of higher cognitive functions arise from larger functional systems whose composition depends on the nature of the task in hand (Luria 1980; Stuss and Benson 1986). In this case the information of interest will be the way in which activity covaries in functionally related brain regions. A more suitable statistical approach would then focus on correlational analyses. The implications of applying different theoretical models of brain function to the analysis of results is discussed in Chap. 6.

## Limitations of the Technique

The tomographic techniques of PET and SPET allow 3-D localization of function within the brain. They represent one avenue of development of the early techniques for visualizing brain function, which measured cortical blood flow using $^{133}$Xe and a relatively small number of fixed surface detectors. This method allowed only limited resolution and imaging was restricted to the cerebral cortex. Progress in SPET and PET technology has improved spatial resolution and enabled the visualization of regions deep within the brain. An alternative avenue of development in cerebral imaging has been followed by Risberg and colleagues (Risberg 1987, 1989). This work has resulted in the production of high-resolution measurements of regional cerebral blood flow which, unlike PET and SPET, are 2-D and restricted to the cortical mantle. The recording system, called the Cortexplorer, has improved spatial resolution by virtue of the use of 254 scintillation detectors, mounted in a helmet so that each may be independently positioned close to the head. With this system spatial resolution has been improved to about 1 cm, compared to the 3–5 cm resolution of standard 32 detector equipment. However, it is still susceptible to the 'look through' phenomenon that limits the sensitivity of blood flow estimation in ischaemic areas that overlie better perfused regions (Risberg 1987). But with respect to temporal resolution one newly reported Cortexplorer procedure has significant advantages over current SPET and PET neuroimaging. In these latter techniques an activation task must be maintained for a number of minutes, from less than 4 (Lammertsma et al. 1989) to more than 20 (Goldenberg et al. 1987). Hence it is not possible to investigate the temporal sequence of activation using these studies because of this poor temporal resolution (Lang et al. 1988). The image of cerebral activity that is finally obtained represents, within the limits of spatial resolution, a temporal summation of the pattern of blood flow occurring during performance of the task. Yet by using injected gold-195m, which has a half-life of 30 s and which is non-diffusible, it is possible to obtain an image of relative distribution of cortical blood flow, but not absolute flow rates, in just 3 s of task performance. Serial measurements are thus possible with the Cortexplorer after just 30 s and the low radioactivity received allows up to 10 injections in normal volunteers (Risberg 1989). With this advantage it should be possible to untangle components of complex tasks in a way not possible if an activation protocol averages cerebral activity over several minutes.

Another potential difficulty is that because SPET provides a functional rather than a structural image, strict anatomical localization of the regions visualized may be problematic (Mazziotta and Phelps 1984). At some specialist centres, software programs are being developed that allow colour SPET or PET images to be superimposed on black and white cranial magnetic resonance images of the same patient, allowing precise anatomic localization. A less sophisticated method of anatomic localization involves identifying brain structures in a SPET image slice from the appropriate slice in the Talairach stereotactic atlas (Talairach and Szilka 1967).

# Summary

When planning a SPET neuroactivation study the following issues must be considered:

1. What results are required?
   a. The cerebral locus of a particular behaviour.
   b. An understanding of the constituent processes that contribute to a complex behaviour.
   These questions have implications for the choice of control and activation tasks and the statistical approach used in the final data analysis.

2. What technology is available/appropriate? If there is no choice, then the study must be constructed bearing in mind the properties of these resources. If a choice is available, then consider the tracer kinetics most suitable for the activation task and subsequent image aquisition.
3. Scan conditions.
   a. If using HMPAO, are the two scans performed close together in time or after radioactivity has decayed following the first scan? Is the dose equally divided between the two scans?
   b. Reliable positioning of the subject.
4. The nature of the control and activation tasks.
   a. Will the activation task actually cause a detectable change in local cerebral activity?
   b. Does the control task match all but the critical feature of the activation task?
   c. Can performance of the tasks be objectively monitored?
   d. Can performance of the tasks be maintained over the period of tracer deposition?
   e. Does the protocol generate reproducible results?
5. The approach used in data analysis.
   a. If ROIs are used, are they drawn reliably, reproducibly and blind to the task condition?
   b. Will discrete changes between regions or correlations between regional changes be sought?
   c. Will statistical corrections be made if multiple comparisons are made?
   d. Can the observed effects be reliably located in the brain, for instance by using superimposed structural images or by reference to a stereotactic atlas?

# References

Andersen AR, Friberg HH, Schmidt JF, et al (1988) Quantitative measurements of cerebral blood flow using SPECT and $^{99m}$Tc-D,L-HMPAO compared to xenon-133. J Cereb Blood Flow Metab 8:S69–S81

Andreasen NC (1988) Evaluation of brain imaging techniques in mental illness. Annual Rev Med 39:335–345

Batjer HH, Devous MD, Meyer MJ, et al (1988) Cerebrovascular haemodynamics in arteriovenous malformation complicated by normal perfusion pressure breakthrough. Neurosurgery 22:503–509

Battisstin L, Pizzolato G, Dam M, et al (1989) Single-photon emission computed tomography studies with 99m-Tc-hexamethylpropyleneamine oxime in dementia: effects of acute administration of L-acetylcarnitine. Eur Neurol 29:261–265

Biersack HJ, Linke D, Brassel F, et al (1987) Technetium-99m HMPAO brain SPECT in epileptic patients before and during unilateral hemispheric anesthesia (Wada test): report of three cases. J Nucl Med 28:1763–1767

Chollet F, Celsis P, Clanet M, et al (1989) SPECT study of cerebral blood flow reactivity after acetazolamide in patients with transient ischaemic attacks. Stroke 20:458–464

Costa DC, Ell PJ, Cullum ID, et al (1986) The in vivo distribution of $^{99}$Tc$^m$-HMPAO in normal man. Nuclear Med Comm 7:647–658

Dahl A, Russel D, Nyberg-Hansen R, et al (1989) Effect of nitroglycerin on cerebral circulation measured by transcranial Doppler and SPECT. Stroke 20:1733–1736

Delecluse F, Voordecker P, Raftopoulos C (1989) Vertebrobasilar insufficiency revealed by xenon-133 inhalation SPECT. Stroke 20:952–956

Ginsberg MD, Yoshii F, Vibulsresth S, et al (1987) Human task-specific somatosensory activation. Neurology 37:1301–1308

Goldenberg G, Podreka I, Steiner M, et al (1987) Patterns of regional cerebral blood flow related to memorizing of high and low imagery words – an emission computer tomography study. Neuropsychologia 25:473–485

Goldenberg G, Podreka I, Uhl F, et al (1989) Cerebral correlates of imagining colours, faces and a map. I. SPECT of regional cerebral blood flow. Neuropsychologia 27:1315–1328

Lammertsma AA, Frackowiak RSJ, Hoffman JM, et al (1989) The C1502 build-up technique to measure regional cerebral blood-flow and volume of distribution of water. J Cereb Blood Flow Metab 9:461–470

Lang W, Lang M, Podreka I, et al (1988) DC-potential shifts and regional cerebral blood flow reveal frontal cortex involvement in human visuomotor learning. Exp Brain Res 71:353–364

Lassen NA, Ingvar DH, Skinhoj E (1978) Brain function and blood flow. Sci Am 239:62–71

Lassen NA, Andersen AR, Friberg L, et al (1988) The retention of [99mTc]-D,L-HMPAO in the human brain after intracarotid bolus injection: a kinetic analysis. J Cereb Blood Flow Metab 8 [Suppl 1]:S13–S22

Luria AR (1980) Higher cortical functions in man, 2nd edn. Basic Books, New York

Matsuda H, Higashi S, Asli IN, et al (1988) Evaluation of cerebral collateral circulation by technetium-99m HMPAO brain SPECT during Matas test: report of three cases. J Nucl Med 29:1724–1729

Mazziotta JC, Phelps ME (1984) Human sensory stimulation and deprivation: positron emission tomographic results and strategies. Ann Neurol 15:S50–S60

Mazziotta JC, Phelps ME (1986) Positron emission tomography studies of the brain. In: Phelps M, Mazziotta J, Schelbert H (eds) Positron emission tomography and autoradiography: principles and applications for the brain and heart. Raven Press, New York, pp 493–579

Petersen SE, Fox PT, Posner MI, et al (1988) Positron emission tomographic studies of the cortical anatomy of single-word processing. Nature 331:585–589

Risberg J (1987) Development of high-resolution two-dimensional measurement of regional cerebral blood flow. In: Wade J, Knezevic S, Maximilian VA, Mubrin Z, Prohvnic I (eds) Impact of functional imaging in neurology and psychiatry. Libbey, London, pp 35–43

Risberg J (1989) Regional cerebral blood flow measurements with high temporal and spatial resolution. In: Ottson D, Rostene W (eds) Visualization of brain functions. Wenner-Gren International Symposium Series, vol 53. Macmillan Press, London, pp 153–158

Roland PE, Friberg L (1985) Localization of cortical areas activated by thinking. J Neurophysiol 53:1219–1243

Sharp PF, Smith FW, Gemmell HG, et al (1986) Technetium-99m-HMPAO stereoisomers as potential agents for imaging regional cerebral blood flow. J Nucl Med 27:171–177

Stuss DT, Benson DF (1986) The frontal lobes. Raven Press, New York

Talairach J, Szilka G (1967) Atlas of stereotaxic anatomy of the telencephalon. Masson & Cie, Paris

Walker-Batson D, Wendt JS, Devous MD, et al (1988) A long-term follow-up case study of crossed aphasia assessed by single-photon emission tomography (SPECT), language, and neuropsychological testing. Brain Lang 33:311–322

Weinberger DR, Berman KF, Zee RF (1986) Physiologic dysfunction of prefrontal cortex in schizophrenia: I. Regional cerebral blood flow evidence. Arch Gen Psychiatry 43:114–124

Woods SW, Hegeman IM, Zubal IG, et al (1991) Visual stimulation increases technetium-99m-HMPAO distribution in human visual cortex. J Nucl Med 32:210–215

Chapter 8
# Review of Previous SPET Neuroactivation Studies in Normal Controls

## Introduction

There are as yet very few SPET activation studies in the published literature. In part, this is because in the first instance functional neuroimaging was used to image the human brain at rest in health and disease. It was only when the technique was familiar and when the appearance of the brain at rest was known that attempts were made to investigate how these appearances changed when the brain received some sort of additional stimulus. Additionally, activation studies make greater demands on the versatility of radioactive ligands and data processing, and until recently most research efforts in these fields have been applied to positron emission tomography (PET).

## Recent Studies

Recently, several SPET activation studies have been published. An investigation of stroboscopic stimulation of the visual cortex was performed to examine the concerns that technetium-99m hexamethylpropylene amine oxime ($^{99m}$Tc-HMPAO) may underestimate regional cerebral blood flow (rCBF) in high rCBF regions (Woods et al. 1991). This activation task was chosen because it was known from previous PET studies that it evoked approximately a 30% increase in visual cortex rCBF. The study involved seven healthy volunteers and the authors followed a protocol that required control and test scans to be separated by a week. On each occasion the subjects received the large dose of 740 MBq of $^{99m}$Tc-HMPAO. The two conditions were chosen to maximize the difference between them, hence the control task consisted of visual deprivation for 6 min. Great attention was paid to accurate repositioning of the head between the two scans, but even so it was not possible to perform an accurate pixel-by-pixel subtraction of the control from the task image. Instead, a region of interest (ROI) analysis was performed using two ROIs, one over the striate cortex and a control region in the left superior temporal/inferior parietal area. The analysis was performed on five successive transaxial slices near and slightly above the level of the basal ganglia, which were identified as containing an area corresponding to the visual cortex by comparison to a brain atlas. It is noted that even in this control area there was a peak increase during activation of 13% in one subject. The authors note the difficulty of eliminating 'noise' from the results and suggest that in this case it may be due to uncontrolled differences in the imaging environment. In the visual cortex the region was a rectangular area centred around the single pixel of maximal percentage increase on activation. The authors acknowledge that basing their calculations on determining the peak change may bias the results towards a more positive finding, but they conclude that the study successfully demonstrates significant activation of the visual cortex by a peak amount of 38%. They infer that $^{99m}$Tc-HMPAO was an appropriate tracer for the study and that comparison with an analogous PET study gave no evidence that it underestimated the increase in rCBF.

While the above study was performed to investigate the methodology involved in SPET activation, other studies have sought to use the technique to explore human cognitive abilities. Goldenberg and colleagues in a series of papers have investigated both memory and cerebral correlates of visual imagery (Goldenberg et al. 1987, 1989a,b). In particular, they wished to determine whether the introspective experience of having mental images corresponded to a distinct mode of cognitive processing. In their first study, using $^{123}$I-N-isopropylamphetamine ($^{123}$IMP) they examined the role of imagery in memorizing abstract and concrete nouns. Because it takes 20 min for the cerebral distribution of the tracer to reach steady-state, the activation task had to be maintained for this period. Hence the maintenance of attention through the task becomes a major issue. In order to examine the effects of such tasks, the resting and memory protocols were generally performed in different subjects, each individual only being scanned in one condition. The comparison of different cerebral states in different brains raises a new group of potential errors since it is not possible to be sure that baseline cerebral states are similar. Additionally, unless all brains are normalized to the same volume (Friston et al. 1989) comparisons between different subjects will be inaccurate because of the difficulties in ensuring that identical brain regions are compared across subjects. However, analysis was also performed within each condition. In this case smallest space analysis was applied to study the pattern of correlations between multiple ROIs within each of the conditions. It was found that all memory tasks involved the hippocampi and inferior temporal regions bilaterally. When an instruction to use imagery was added to the conditions, increased activity was noted in the superior and middle frontal gyri. The authors then applied their results to the more general psychological debate over hemisphere specialization. Prior to the advent of functional neuroimaging evidence of regional and hemisphere specialization was based on the study of subjects with focal brain lesions and absent or sectioned corpus callosum. While such studies have produced a large body of knowledge that is applied to the workings of the intact brain, the new activation techniques allow the investigation of cerebral localization directly in healthy brains. Hence there is no danger that the presence of focal pathology will confound the results obtained.

In subsequent studies of the cerebral correlates of various forms of visual imagery the same group used a different study protocol. In this case all subjects were scanned twice, once at rest and once during the performance of an imaging task. The tracer used was $^{99m}$Tc-HMPAO, allowing a shortening of the time for which the activation task was maintained. The studies were arranged so that complementary hypotheses regarding the role of visual imagery in solving cognitive problems could be tested. Evidence was collected that imagery is selectively related to the activity of inferior-temporal and occipital regions but that the exact cerebral localization depends on what kind of information is being depicted, as well as on the cognitive nature of the task. In addition, further studies examined the role of the information content of the image to be visualized and the nature of the image. While overall information quantity, as measured by comparing the imagining of a single colour field to a face or a spatial map, resulted in difference in rCBF, the nature of the information, facial versus spatial, did not affect response.

Lange et al. (1988) investigated the rCBF changes associated with visuomotor learning in normal volunteers. The task involved learning to track a moving target across a screen, applying a rule of horizontal inversion (left becomes right and right becomes left). The control task required simply straightforward tracking of the target. These tasks appear well chosen in that all the visual and motor components are matched, leaving only the learning and application of the inversion rule to produce differences in the two conditions. The methodology used in the study resembled that in the latter two studies described above. The tracer utilized was $^{99m}$Tc-HMPAO, each subject was scanned twice, once for each condition, and the two scans were performed between 7 and 14 days apart. Data analysis involved the measurement of activity in multiple regions of interest. However, unlike the studies reported by Goldenberg and colleagues, in this work as well as looking for correlations in changing activities between regions, individual regional differences in the ROIs between the regions were compared using Student's *t*-test. This approach assumes that the values of different regions are independent of one another. The authors justify this position by stating that they are testing the a priori hypothesis that the frontal lobe is critically involved in the performance of the activation task. However, the correlational analysis that was also performed revealed a correlation between ipsilateral medial frontal and parietal areas. Hence although the authors conclude that their study supports the hypothesis that the frontal lobe plays an important role in visuomotor learning, this conclusion seems to neglect the possible role of a coordinated frontal-parietal functional structure.

# Conclusion

In summary, it appears that activation studies in normal volunteers have a role both in examining the methodologies involved in such studies and also in the examination of the cerebral processes underlying human cognitive tasks. However, it is also clear that the results obtained, as well as the interpretation placed on these results, is highly dependent on the scan protocols and the data analysis techniques employed.

# References

Friston KJ, Passingham RE, Nutt JG, et al (1989) Localization in PET images: direct fitting of the intercommissural (AC-PC) line. J Cereb Blood Flow Metab 9:690–695

Goldenberg G, Podreka I, Steiner M, et al (1987) Patterns of regional cerebral blood flow related to memorizing of high and low imagery words – an emission computer tomography study. Neuropsychologia 25:473–485

Goldenberg G, Podreka I, Uhl F, et al (1989a) Cerebral correlates of imagining colours, faces and a map, I. SPECT of regional cerebral blood flow. Neuropsychologia 27:1315–1328

Goldenberg G, Podreka I, Steiner M, et al (1989b) Regional cerebral blood flow patterns in visual imagery. Neuropsychologia 27:641–664

Lang W, Lang M, Podreka I, et al (1988) DC-potential shifts and regional cerebral blood flow reveal frontal cortex involvement in human visuomotor learning. Exp Brain Res 71:353–364

Woods SW, Hegeman IM, Zubal IG, et al (1991) Visual stimulation increases technetium-99m-HMPAO distribution in human visual cortex. J Nucl Med 32:210–215

Chapter 9

# Activation Protocols in Normal Subjects Using SPET: A Window into Normal Brain Function

## Introduction

In previous chapters we described the principles of neuroactivation and reviewed the previous studies of SPET neuroactivation in normal controls. In this chapter we describe several neuroactivation procedures developed by the authors at the UCMSM Institute of Nuclear Medicine using the Neurocam, a high-sensitivity and high-resolution SPET system described in Chap. 3. These activation protocols were designed to explore motor, cognitive and sensory tasks.

## Methods

During each activation protocol described below we used basically the same imaging parameters and the same time-frame for scanning.

Please refer to Fig. 1. For the first scan (the control, C) subjects were placed in the control environment with the control conditions. Two minutes into this control environment they were given intravenous technetium-99m hexamethylpropylene amine oxime ($^{99m}$Tc-HMPAO) (5 MBq/kg average) and remained under the same conditions for another 4 min. They were then scanned supine for approximately 15 min (128 projections in a 64 × 64 matrix acquisition) using high-resolution collimators. Immediately after the first scan they were reseated under the same conditions as before, except that they performed the task (T) behaviour for 6 min. $^{99m}$Tc-HMPAO (5 MBq/kg average) was administered 2 min into this procedure (the task, T) and subjects were rescanned, as before, with their heads in the same position. Tomographic slices were then reconstructed in the transaxial, coronal and sagittal planes using a Hanning prefilter with 1.0 cycles/cm cut-off frequency, a Ramp filter and attenuation correction.

For each subject, brain regions of interest (ROI) were analysed after

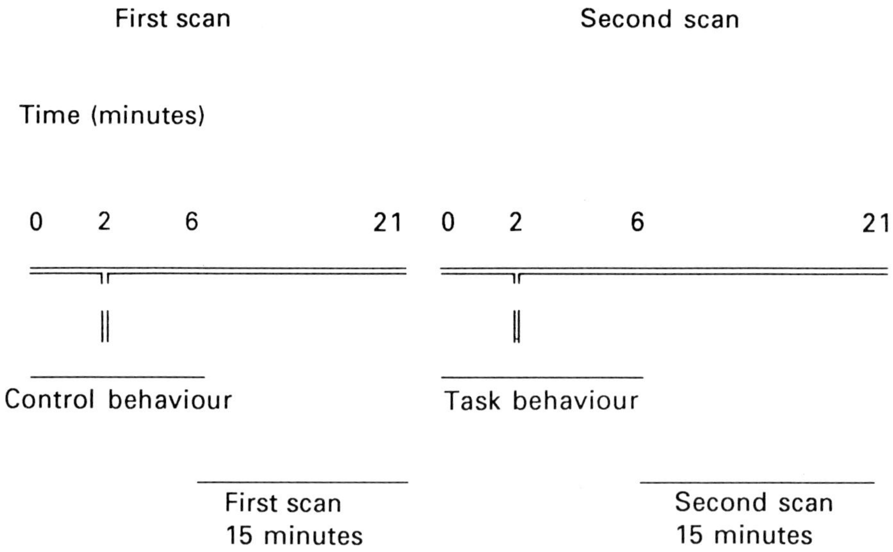

```
            First scan                        Second scan

Time (minutes)

 0    2      6              21      0    2      6              21
 ═════╤╤═════════════════════       ═════╤╤═════════════════════
      ‖                                  ‖
 ─────────────────                  ─────────────────
 Control behaviour                  Task behaviour

        ─────────────────                  ─────────────────
            First scan                          Second scan
            15 minutes                          15 minutes
```

**Fig 1.** Diagram of the time course of the activation protocols reviewed in this chapter. $^{99m}$Tc-HMPAO is injected at time 2 min into each behaviour (C or T). In the optimal activation protocol there is no delay between the first and second scan.

normalizing the two scans (C and T) to the same total number of brain counts. This is done by summing the total number of counts on the planar projection images for the C and T scans and computing the conversion factor = (task scan total counts)/(control scan total counts). Then the control images are multiplied by this conversion factor to obtain the normalized images. Using $4 \times 4$ pixel regions ($1.6 \times 1.6$ cm$^2$ brain area) and ROI analysis, the percent activation for each brain region can be calculated by the following formula: % activation = $(T-C)/ 0.5(T+C)$. The ROI analysis can be done in several ways. First, the control scans can be analysed, followed sequentially by the task scans. Second, using a split-screen approach, the same image from each scan (C and T) can be displayed side by side, and ROI analysis can be obtained. The calculated activity in each region is the average of three independent samples on three different slices. Third, alternatively, when the images are subtracted pixel-by-pixel, the net activated area can be represented as a separate image. ROI analysis can then be computed on this activated area. ROI sampling methods 1 and 2 have 1.5% coefficient of variation in these sampled regions for test/retest reliability.

# Motor Tasks

As we reviewed in Chap. 5, over 130 years ago David Ferrier electrically stimulated the premotor cortex in animals and produced contralateral limb movement. Since that time, the concept of a cortical map of human movement

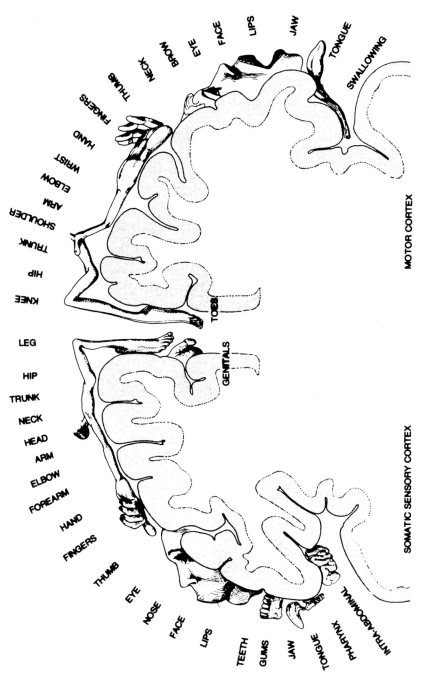

**Fig 2.** Diagrams of the human motor (*right*) and sensory (*left*) homunculus.

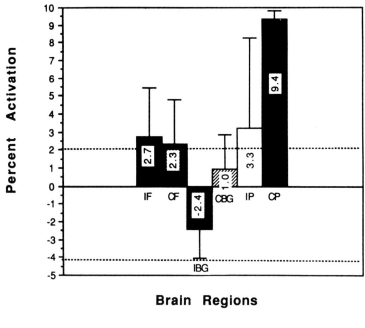

IF = Ipsilateral frontal  
CF = Contralateral frontal  
IBG = Ipsilateral basal ganglia  
CBG = Contralateral basal ganglia  
IP = Ipsilateral parietal  
CP = Contralateral parietal  

**Fig 3.** SPET regional percent activation of four subjects performing a finger-opposition task. Average percent activation for different brain regions with standard errors of the mean (SEM) are shown. The *two dotted lines* (+2.1 to −4.2%) represent the regional brain activity range (2 standard deviations, 95% confidence interval) on two subjects using this technique without an activation task. Note the wide SEM for the ipsilateral parietal cortex, possibly demonstrating mirror activation.

has been reinforced by lesion studies, electrophysiological studies, electrical stimulation during neurosurgery and PET studies. Most studies support the idea of a contralateral cortical homunculus similar to Fig. 2.

In order to investigate whether high-resolution SPET might demonstrate parietal activation we studied four normal volunteers twice (all right-handed, 2M, 2F, average age 36 [25–65]) on the triple-headed brain-dedicated SPET system, the GE/CGR Neurocam, described in Chap. 3.

## Parietal Lobe Activation

For the first scan (the control, C), subjects were seated and resting with minimal movement in a quiet room, with their ears and eyes open looking at a blank wall. Immediately after the first scan they were reseated under the same conditions as before, except using one hand they alternately opposed their thumb to their other digits in a sequential manner (finger-opposition task, T)

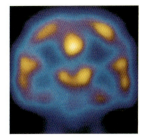 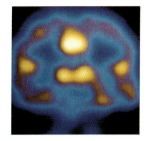 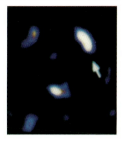

**Fig 4.** Coronal SPET images of one subject during control conditions (*left*), then performing a finger opposition task (*middle*), with the subtracted image (T-C) (*right*) demonstrating activation of the contralateral parietal cortex.

for 6 min. To assess whether dominance mattered for activation, three subjects used their dominant (right) hand, while one subject used his left.

## Results

The average percent activation for each brain region is shown in Fig. 3. The average activation of the contralateral parietal lobe in this study was 9.4% (range 8.7–10.9, standard error of the mean 0.5). Figure 4 displays an image generated by subtracting, pixel-by-pixel, the task from the control scan. ROI analysis of the circumscribed activated area in Fig. 4 reveals a 14.5% average activation. Our results correspond with previous electrophysiological, PET and electrical stimulation studies demonstrating contralateral parietal lobe involvement in fine motor movements (Penfield and Rasmussen 1950; Kandel and Schwartz 1981). Interestingly, two subjects showed possible mirror activation of the ipsilateral parietal cortex, reflected in the wide standard error of the mean for this region. This SPET activation technique demonstrated neuronal activation during a motor task.

## Discussion

This neuroactivation protocol was chosen because of its simplicity in order to demonstrate that high-resolution SPET, combined with $^{99m}$Tc-HMPAO, can demonstrate neuroactivation. As we reviewed in Chap. 8, previous SPET activation protocols required subjects to have their scans separated by 2 weeks. This obviously introduces a host of variables that may affect the scans. Our same-day protocol eliminates this fortnight delay: the actual activation takes 6 min, followed by 15 min of scanning, so the delay between the control and task scans is theoretically only 27 min (6+15+6). Therefore, variables such as time from the last meal or from taking a medication can be minimized. This parietal neuroactivation protocol, now that it has been shown to work in controls, is being applied to patients with disease states such as strokes or movement disorders. These applications are discussed in Chap. 10.

## Form C Stimulus Sheet

| | | | |
|---|---|---|---|
| BLUE | RED | TAN | RED |
| GREEN | GREEN | RED | TAN |
| TAN | TAN | TAN | RED |
| RED | BLUE | BLUE | TAN |
| GREEN | GREEN | TAN | BLUE |
| BLUE | BLUE | RED | GREEN |
| GREEN | TAN | GREEN | RED |
| BLUE | GREEN | RED | BLUE |
| RED | TAN | BLUE | RED |
| BLUE | BLUE | TAN | TAN |
| TAN | GREEN | RED | GREEN |
| RED | BLUE | GREEN | TAN |
| TAN | GREEN | RED | BLUE |
| GREEN | RED | TAN | RED |
| BLUE | BLUE | BLUE | BLUE |
| TAN | GREEN | TAN | RED |
| GREEN | TAN | GREEN | GREEN |
| RED | RED | TAN | RED |
| TAN | TAN | BLUE | BLUE |
| RED | GREEN | TAN | TAN |
| TAN | TAN | BLUE | BLUE |
| RED | RED | GREEN | GREEN |
| GREEN | BLUE | RED | BLUE |
| RED | RED | GREEN | RED |
| TAN | GREEN | TAN | BLUE |
| BLUE | RED | RED | TAN |
| GREEN | TAN | GREEN | BLUE |
| TAN | BLUE | BLUE | GREEN |

**Fig 5 A,B.** Two different versions of the Stroop task used in a frontal activation task. **A** The black and white control of the Stroop task and **B** the colour Stroop task.

A

# Form C Stimulus Sheet

| | | | |
|---|---|---|---|
| BLUE | RED | TAN | RED |
| GREEN | GREEN | RED | TAN |
| TAN | TAN | TAN | RED |
| RED | BLUE | BLUE | TAN |
| GREEN | GREEN | TAN | BLUE |
| BLUE | BLUE | RED | GREEN |
| GREEN | TAN | GREEN | RED |
| BLUE | GREEN | RED | BLUE |
| RED | TAN | BLUE | RED |
| BLUE | BLUE | TAN | TAN |
| TAN | GREEN | RED | GREEN |
| RED | BLUE | GREEN | TAN |
| TAN | GREEN | RED | BLUE |
| GREEN | RED | TAN | RED |
| BLUE | BLUE | BLUE | BLUE |
| TAN | GREEN | TAN | RED |
| GREEN | TAN | GREEN | GREEN |
| RED | RED | TAN | RED |
| TAN | TAN | BLUE | BLUE |
| RED | GREEN | TAN | TAN |
| TAN | TAN | BLUE | BLUE |
| RED | RED | GREEN | GREEN |
| GREEN | BLUE | RED | BLUE |
| RED | RED | GREEN | RED |
| TAN | GREEN | TAN | BLUE |
| BLUE | RED | RED | TAN |
| GREEN | TAN | GREEN | BLUE |
| | BLUE | BLUE | GREEN |

B

## Cognitive Tasks

Motor activation of the cortex using SPET is necessary and may prove extremely useful in the management of certain diseases such as stroke and movement disorders. However, to really use SPET neuroactivation to probe the human brain one would like to demonstrate neuroactivation with more complex tasks – tasks that require thinking and planning. Thus cognitive tasks are at once more interesting clinically and for research, but are more difficult to conceive and execute. They may also be more difficult to detect with neuroimaging, as the expected magnitude of rCBF changes with cognitive tasks is lower than with motor tasks (Ginsberg et al. 1987).

## Frontal Lobe Activation

We have used two different activation protocols to probe frontal lobe function.

### The Stroop Protocol

For the first scan (the control, C), subjects were seated and resting in a quiet room with minimal movement with their eyes and ears open. They were instructed to read aloud slowly a black-and-white version of the Stroop sheet (Stroop 1935) (see Fig. 5A). Two minutes later, they were given the first injection and continued to read aloud under the same conditions for another 4 min. Immediately after the first scan they were reseated under the same conditions, except they were instructed to read a colour version of the Stroop (see Fig. 5B). They were instructed to ignore the written word and instead pronounce the colour of the typeface for the word. This requires the active inhibition of pronouncing one word while speaking the colour. The second injection was administered 2 min into this procedure (the task, T) and the subject was rescanned as before with the head in the same position. Tomographic reconstruction and ROI analysis were as described previously.

*Results* Disappointingly, for the two subjects tested in this protocol, no clear activation of the frontal lobes was detected. Figure 6 shows the ROI percentage change for one subject.

*Discussion* There are several possible explanations as to why we did not detect frontal activation using this protocol. The sample size is small, and we might have chosen two subjects who for some reason did not activate. Both of the subjects were postgraduate medical personnel and the task may have been too easy for them. Thus we may have found a type II error due to a small sample size. Alternatively, this protocol may not have been rigorous enough. The task and control environments differed with respect to reading in colour versus reading in black and white. This conceivably could have masked the frontal activation. However, this minor uncontrolled variable seems unlikely to explain our lack of findings totally.

It may be that the Stroop task, although sensitive for patients with frontal

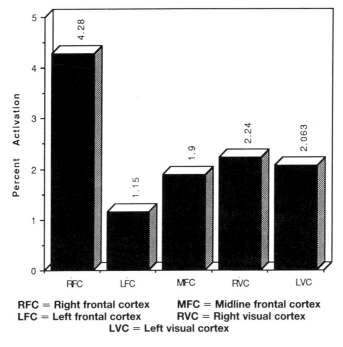

**Fig 6.** Regional percent brain changes in one subject using the Stroop protocol.

lobe damage, does not actually activate the frontal lobes. We saw in Chap. 5 that localizing a lesion is much easier than localizing a function. Functioning frontal lobes are *necessary* to perform the Stroop, but frontal lobes alone are not *sufficient* to carry it out, nor does performing the Stroop activate the frontal lobes in the way that moving one's fingers activates the parietal lobes. Whatever the reason for the lack of frontal activation using the Stroop, in our experience it was not a useful activation protocol.

## The FAS Word-Generation Protocol

In order to demonstrate frontal lobe activation with SPET we recently studied and obtained images from five normal volunteers twice (3 males, 2 females, mean age 30 years) as follows:

For the first scan (control, C), subjects were seated and resting with minimal movement in a quiet room, with their eyes and ears open looking at a blank wall. They were instructed to name out loud, sequentially, the months of the year. They pronounced a new month every 3 s after being prompted by the word 'next'. After doing this for 2 min they were given the first injection. They were then instructed to name the days of the week sequentially in the same manner for 2 min. Finally, they listed the alphabet sequentially under the same conditions and were then scanned. Immediately after the first scan they were

P 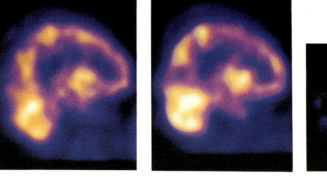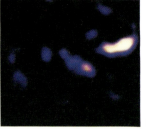 A

**Fig 7.** Sagittal images of a subject during a control behaviour (*left*), generating new words (*middle*) and a subtracted image showing the brain regions activated by the task.

reseated under the same conditions and were asked to generate new words beginning with the letters 'F' for 2 min, followed by 'A' for 2 min, followed by 'S' for 2 min. They were prompted every 3 s to pronounce a new word by the command 'next'. After the first 2 min of the task they were given the second injection. The second scan was performed as before, with the head in the same position. Tomographic reconstruction and ROI analysis were performed as described earlier.

*Results* The average percent activation for the frontal lobes using the ROI analysis method of taking three independent samples from three different slices was: right frontal 0.74% (range 6.8 to − 4.1%), left frontal 1.64% (range 3.5 to −7.0%) and mid-frontal 3.21% (range 6.6 to -3.0%). These results are modest because the method of taking samples from three regions greatly dilutes the activated area with surrounding brain activity. A more precise method of judging activation involves performing ROI analysis over the subtracted images. Subtracting pixel-by-pixel the task from the control scan generates pictures of the brain regions activated by the task in an individual patient (Figs. 7, 8). ROI analysis of these activated regions ranged from 8 to 12%.

*Discussion* The FAS word-generation task is a common clinical screening task for frontal lobe damage and perseveration. However, as was noted with the Stroop test, a screening test for frontal lobe damage will not necessarily activate the brain area in question.

The FAS protocol as outlined above follows most of the principles of neuroactivation. The control setting adequately controls for speech production, hearing the prompt word and storing and remembering what one has previously said. We chose the categories 'months of the year', 'days of the week' and the alphabet because these are, in most people, overlearned categories requiring little effort to generate. Thus, this protocol hopefully isolates the mental effort required to generate new ideas within the same category.

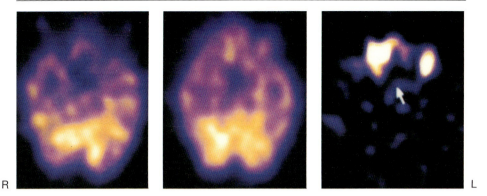

**Fig 8.** Transaxial images of a subject during a control behaviour (*left*), generating new words (*middle*) and a subtracted image showing the brain regions activated by the task.

We speculate whether the way one generates new words determines which part of the frontal lobe is activated by the FAS task, that is, which frontal lobe is activated may depend on the strategy the subject uses to solve the word generation task. Some of the subjects had lexical rules that they followed (e.g. words with Fa..., Fe..., Fi...), whereas others seemed to 'visualize' words, or find new words by category association (e.g. 'farm', 'field', 'fertilizer',...). Our sample size was too small to analyse these differences but this is an intriguing area that needs further study.

Unfortunately, we have not yet reversed the order in which we have people perform the control or task. Thus we are unsure what role anxiety plays in this activation. Early in our work, we scanned two subjects with the same conditions for the first and second scans and found no significant changes in regional flow. In the FAS protocol all subjects were anxious with the first injection and appeared calmer with the task. One would expect that anxiety might increase frontal blood flow, much as it has been demonstrated to increase right parahippocampal blood flow in patients with overwhelming anxiety (panic attacks) (Reiman et al. 1989). Thus, if anything, lower anxiety about the pain of the injection during the task would decrease our frontal lobe results.

This protocol generates questions about other interesting areas. Subjects were asked not to use common names but some did anyway. Does this affect the results? Analysis of our small sample did not find any association. Additionally, two of the subjects spoke English as a second language and did not respond with their first language. Again, we did not find that this greatly influenced the results. Finally, most of the subjects were physicians or ancillary medical personnel. The world of medicine has been said to have its own second language and several subjects freely tapped their medical lexicon (e.g. 'fasciculation', 'festinating',..). We did not find that it affected the results.

Despite these findings, one must be cautious in interpreting these results. Subjects were intelligent and highly motivated to perform the task well. It remains to be seen how well this task works in people with less attention due to a disease process such as depression or dementia. We will discuss potential applications of this protocol in Chap. 10.

## Sensory Tasks

We have shown how SPET neuroimaging with $^{99m}$Tc-HMPAO and a high-resolution system can demonstrate activation during a motor or cognitive task. Another way to state this is that we have shown activation of the frontal lobe and motor cortex. Another extremely interesting area of the brain is the occipital cortex and the complex processes involved with vision (see Fig. 9). Below we describe two activation protocols for the occipital lobes.

## Occipital Lobe Activation (Pursuit)

In order to investigate occipital lobe activation with SPET we studied two normal volunteers (both right-handed males, ages 26 and 27) using the Neurocam. For the first scan subjects were seated and resting with minimal movement in a quiet darkened room, with their eyes and ears open. The subjects were instructed to stare at a small (4 mm) blue dot on a pink wall 1.5 m in front of them. They were instructed not to move their eyes away from the dot. Two minutes into this procedure they were given the first injection and continued staring without moving their eyes for another 4 min. They were then scanned. Immediately after the first scan they were reseated under the

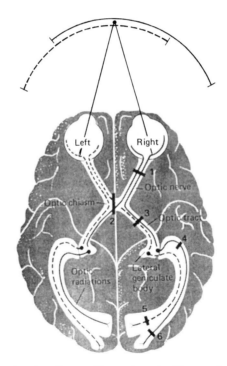

**Fig 9.** Diagram of the visual pathway. (Reproduced with permission from Kandel and Schwarz, 1981).

P 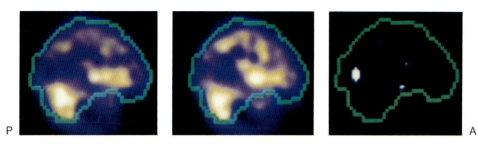 A

**Fig 10.** Sagittal SPET images of a subject staring at a fixed spot on the wall (*left*), following a beam of light (*middle*) and a subtracted image showing the brain regions activated by this task.

same conditions as before. For the task they were instructed to follow with their eyes a moving light beam which randomly moved in straight or diagonal patterns between dots fixed in a 1.5 m by 1 m rectangle on the wall in front of the patient. The light beam moved on average 2 dots/s. Two minutes into this procedure the second injection was administered, the procedure continued for another 4 min and the subject was rescanned as before, with the head in the same position. Tomographic reconstruction and ROI analysis were performed as discussed earlier.

## Results

Figures 10 and 11 show the activated regions generated by subtracting the control from the task scans. ROI analysis in these regions showed on average 10% activation.

## Discussion

This visual activation task robustly demonstrates activation of the occipital lobes. It remains to be seen whether it is the processing of different images (squares, diagonals, etc.) or the motor task of following a light that activates these lateral occipital regions. The process of following an object is controlled by the occipital cortex, whereas voluntary eye movements are controlled by the frontal eye fields (Adams and Victor 1989). We chose this task in order to avoid activating the frontal fields. We describe next a voluntary eye movement protocol that activates this relatively small area and the frontal lobes. Different neurons in the occipital cortex respond to certain visual stimuli, depending on the pattern. We chose a random pattern that would generate diagonal, horizontal and vertical lines in an attempt to activate as many of these occipital cells as possible. Future work using a protocol similar to this one could attempt to locate specific areas of the visual cortex involved in processing specific types of stimuli.

Visual tasks, more than other neuroactivation procedures, require strict consideration of the many variables that may influence the activation.

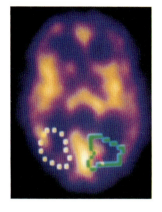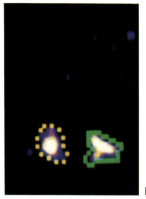

**Fig 11.** Transaxial SPET images of a subject staring at a fixed spot (*left*), following a beam of light (*middle*) and a subtracted image showing the brain regions activated.

## Occipital Lobe Activation (Voluntary Eye Movements)

In one volunteer we carried out the following protocol. For the first scan the subject was seated and resting with minimal movement in a quiet room, with eyes and ears open. The subject was instructed to stare, without looking away, at a small (30 mm) number '2' on a pink wall 1.5 m in front of her. A stopwatch beeped aloud every second. For the task behaviour, the subject was instructed to look at the wall in front of her, where the numbers 1–6 were posted in a random pattern forming a rectangle. The subject was instructed to move her eyes each second when she heard the beep, and focus on the numbers in order (i.e. 1,2,3,...).

*Results*

Figure 12 demonstrates the areas activated by this task in this subject. ROI analysis of these regions shows an average 12% activation.

*Discussion*

This task appears to involve frontal, basal ganglia and occipital regions. Further protocols to dissect out the various aspects of this task will help isolate which areas of the brain are involved in this task.

## Conclusion

We have reviewed above how $^{99m}$Tc-HMPAO SPET can be used to demonstrate the activation of specific brain regions during differing tasks. This technology can be used to help us understand, like never before, how the human mind and brain act to produce behaviour. In addition to probing the

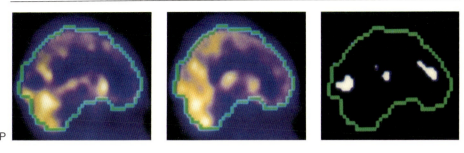

P                                                      A

**Fig 12.** Sagittal images of a subject during a control behaviour (*left*), performing a voluntary eye movement task (*middle*) and the subtracted image of activated areas (*right*).

healthy brain, activation protocols such as the ones demonstrated above can also be used to investigate disease. We turn to this interesting area in the next chapter.

# References

Adams RD, Victor M (1989) Principles of neurology, 4th edn. McGraw Hill, New York
Ginsberg MD, Yoshii F, Vibulsresth S, et al (1987) Human task-specific somatosensory activation. Neurology 37:1301–1308
Kandel ER, Schwartz JH (1981) Principles of neural science. Elsevier/North Holland, New York, p 324
Penfield W, Rasmussen T (1950) The cerebral cortex of man. Macmillan, New York
Reiman EM, Fusselman MS, Fox PT, et al (1989) Neuroanatomical correlates of/anticipatory/ anxiety. Science 243:1071–1074
Stroop JR (1935) Studies of interference in serial verbal reactions. J Exp Psychol 18:643–662

Chapter 10
# Activation Studies in Specific Disease States: Future Applications

## Introduction

In Chap. 9 we reviewed the exciting potential of SPET neuroactivation for understanding how the brain works in healthy controls. Despite this potential for studying normal brain function, SPET may possibly lag behind PET in this area over the next decade for several reasons. First, it is usually easier to label biologically active compounds with a radioactive carbon, nitrogen, fluoride or oxygen atom than it is to label them with single photon emitters such as $^{99m}$Tc or $^{123}$I. Additionally, the shorter physical half-life of the tracers used in PET allow multiple images (6–10) to be taken of the same subject in a single activation session, thus increasing the statistical power to detect subtle functional changes. Of course, these are countered by the expense and relative non-availability of PET as we saw in Chaps. 1 and 2.

But because of these reasons, the real future importance of SPET neuroactivation may perhaps lie in the area of activating specific functions in diseased patients in order to help in their diagnosis, treatment and recovery. In this clinical realm, with wide-spread availability and relatively low costs per scan, SPET neuroactivation may perhaps find an important clinical niche. In this chapter we review the published studies where SPET neuroactivation has been used to probe neuropsychiatric disease. We also report on several neuroactivation studies under way at the Institute of Nuclear Medicine at UCMSM. As we review these studies we sketch possible future clinical and research uses of SPET neuroactivation.

## Review of Previous SPET Activation Studies in Disease

Because the technology of SPET neuroactivation is extremely new, there are few published studies using SPET neuroactivation in various diseases (see

Table 1. SPET activation studies in neuropsychiatric diseases

| Study | Question | Activation | Control |
|---|---|---|---|
| *Dementia* | | | |
| Battistin et al. (1989) | Effect of L-acetyl carnitine on rCBF in Alzheimer's | Injection of L-acetylcarnitine | Pre-injection awake, quiet, eyes closed |
| *Epilepsy* | | | |
| Biersack et al. (1987) | Effect of hemisphere anaesthesia on rCBF with respect to speech dominance and epileptic focus | Unilateral hemisphere anaesthesia | Pre-injection 'routine SPET' |
| *Cerebrovascular disease* | | | |
| Matsuda et al. (1988) | Efficacy of brain collateral circulation | Unilateral carotid occlusion | No occlusion |
| Chollet et al. (1989) | Are there changes in cerebrovascular reactivity after TIAs? | Injection of 1 g acetazolamide | Rest pre-injection |
| Delecluse et al. (1989) | Are there changes in cerebrovascular reactivity associated with vertebrobasilar insufficiency? | Injection of 1 g acetazolamide | Rest pre-injection |

Table 1). For many behaviours, the necessary groundwork with controls has not been completed. Generally, before studying an activation procedure in a group of diseased patients, one must be sure that the task activates the brain area in question. Currently there have only been sporadic reports of SPET activation studies in normal controls (see Chaps. 8 and 9). These have utilized varying test paradigms and different methods of data analysis in different patient populations. In such circumstances it is difficult to validate techniques for performing activation studies that will allow these normative findings to be used in studies of individual patients with differing conditions. The lack of clinical studies will certainly not last long, however, as clinicians and researchers begin to realize the power of this new technique. In the future it may be that the development of a data bank based on the use of 'standard' techniques across a range of subjects will increase the power of observations made in individual cases.

## Cerebrovascular Disease

Because SPET can directly provide information about blood flow to the brain (rCBF), it lends itself particularly well to evaluating patients with cerebrovascular disease. There have been at least three published studies where two SPET scans have been separated by a measure designed to change the brain (activate) and provide information about cerebrovascular reactivity.

Matsuda et al. (1988) used $^{99m}$Tc-HMPAO SPET to study the efficacy of collateral circulation in the pre-surgical work-up of patients with intracranial aneurysms. For the first scan patients were scanned at rest. During the second scan the patients were injected 30 s after the beginning of unilateral carotid occlusion. They were thus able to measure rCBF in each hemisphere pre- and post-unilateral carotid occlusion.

There was a 19% average decrease in rCBF on the affected hemisphere with carotid occlusion. Two other studies used as their 'task' the injection of 1 g of acetazolamide, a potent vasodilator. Using SPET and this drug challenge, the authors in these two studies sought to investigate the vascular reactivity of patients with cerebrovascular disease. Chollet et al. (1989) imaged 15 patients within 1 month after a transient ischaemic attack (TIA). Normal rCBF SPET studies (not using a drug challenge) had shown hypoperfused areas in 40% of TIA patients. Seven of the TIA patients showed a focal hypoperfusion at rest in the appropriate hemisphere for their symptoms (agreeing with the previous studies). Seven other TIA patients whose resting studies were normal, showed hyporeactive areas after acetazolamide administration. Thus, with activation of acetazolamide, 14/15 patients with TIAs had areas of hypoperfusion that correlated with their TIA symptoms. The use of a cortical neuroactivator, acetazolamide, greatly increased the sensitivity of SPET for detecting functional evidence of recent TIAs.

In a similar report of one case, Delecluse et al. (1989) demonstrated impaired occipital rCBF response (vertebrobasilar insufficiency) to acetazolamide in a patient with hypertension and attacks of nausea and vertigo. Three weeks later the patient suffered an extensive ischaemic stroke in the areas of impaired rCBF previously demonstrated by SPET.

In summary, one sees that SPET neuroactivation holds great promise in the area of clinical cerebrovascular disease.

## Schizophrenia

One of the more interesting and possibly frustrating diseases to study with SPET may be schizophrenia. Using SPET, researchers may begin to tease apart certain subgroups of the schizophrenias that will allow refinement of both treatment and research. Although it was not technically an activation protocol, Musalek et al. (1988) used $^{99m}$Tc-HMPAO SPET to examine the effects on regional cerebral blood flow of auditory and tactile hallucinations in patients with schizophrenia. Unfortunately, the authors of this study compared their patients to a normal control group instead of rescanning each patient after they were no longer hallucinating. They thus failed to control for the non-hallucinatory features of mental illness. More precise results might have been obtained from scanning the same patients both in and out of an hallucinatory period. The power of SPET neuroactivation in this area could have been used if the same subjects had been scanned twice, once while hallucinating and a second time when they were free of hallucinations but listening to external sounds similar to their hallucinations. SPET in this situation could have revealed information both about schizophrenia and cerebral function during hallucinations. By analysing this study and reformulating it in a way that incorporates neuroactivation principles, one sees the power of this new technology.

Notardonato et al. (1989) reported on a patient with auditory hallucinations who had iodine-123 iodoamphetamine ($^{123}$I-IMP) SPET scans before and after pharmacological treatment and improvement. The initial scan showed focally increased tracer uptake in the caudate nuclei and the right temporal lobe, which resolved with treatment. Again, had the authors instructed the patient to listen to an external reproduction of the hallucinations, interesting information could have been learned about the cerebral processing of hallucinations.

Using the word 'activation' in a broad sense, there is current ongoing work at UCMSM looking at changes in brain function in patients with schizophrenia on and off medication. Using a specific D2 ligand, iodobenzamide (IBZM), Pilowski et al. (1991) are studying changes in dopamine function pre- and post-treatment with a dopamine-blocking agent.

A number of SPET studies have correlated functional images of pathological states with test scores describing the clinical state of the patient (Hunter et al. 1989; Homan et al. 1989). However, changes observed within an activation protocol may also be correlated with clinical scores. In a deoxyglucose PET scan study of chronic schizophrenia, Volkow et al. (1987) correlated a clinical score of disease severity with cerebral global and frontal metabolic rates at rest and in a smooth pursuit eye tracking activation task. It was found that the more severely affected patients failed to show a change in metabolic activity on activation. The authors concluded that cerebral metabolic patterns reflected the clinical characteristics of these patients. Although in this particular study there were confounding variables, such as different drug treatment regimes for the more and the less sick, the study demonstrates the potential value of correlating clinical scores with different test conditions to allow better understanding of the clinical significance of rCBF changes during activation.

These studies demonstrate how SPET neuroactivation may play an important role in advancing our understanding of schizophrenia.

## Epilepsy

In Chap. 4 we reviewed the clinical importance of SPET in the evaluation of epilepsy patients with focal seizures. Lang et al. (1988) used 'neuroactivation' to study focal blood flow changes associated with a seizure. They compared patterns of brain activity in three epileptic patients during a seizure, 3–7 days after the seizure and then again 2–6 weeks later using SPET. They were thus able to follow in the same patient the transition from increased to decreased relative blood flow in the region of the focus. We reviewed in Chap. 4 how Bajc et al. (1989) scanned patients with SPET during and after electroconvulsive therapy (ECT), finding increased activity in the frontal, frontotemporal and basal ganglia regions during the iatrogenically produced convulsions. The therapeutic mechanism of action of ECT is unknown. SPET studies such as this may help unravel this enigma.

A further example of the creative use of SPET in understanding epilepsy is illustrated in the following example. A 25-year-old man with cortical myoclonus, mostly left-sided, was studied and scanned three times using $^{99m}$Tc-HMPAO: (1) resting, (2) with electrical stimulation of his right leg, and (3) with electrical stimulation of his left leg (see Fig. 1). This same principle could be

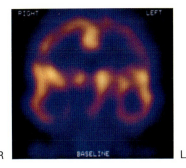
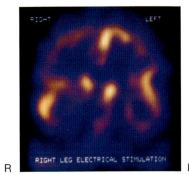
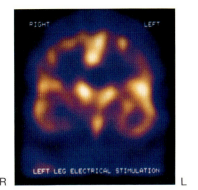

**Fig 1.** SPET scans of a patient with cortical myoclonus. The images were taken at rest (*top*), while receiving electrical stimulation of his right leg (*middle*) and while receiving electrical stimulation of his left leg (*bottom*). Note the increased activity in the left parietal region with right-sided stimulation. The same stimulation on the affected side (the patient's left) does not produce the same increase in cortical activity in the contralateral right hemisphere (*bottom*).

used to study the reflex epilepsies, where specific activities (e.g. reading, singing, listening to music) cause seizures.

Another interesting application of SPET neuroactivation in the evaluation of epilepsy was demonstrated by Biersack et al. (1987). They used $^{99m}$Tc-HMPAO to study three patients with temporal lobe epilepsy who were candidates for possible temporal lobectomy. Perhaps this should be called SPET 'neuroinactivation' as SPET scans were obtained before and during unilateral anaesthesia of one hemisphere to determine lateralization of speech dominance. The authors found a 10–45% decrease of rCBF during anaesthesia, with the dominant hemisphere showing a much greater change. Clearly there are interesting possible uses of SPET neuroactivation that may help us understand the epilepsies.

## Parkinson's Disease

One obvious use of SPET neuroactivation in the study of Parkinson's disease is to study patients on and off medications. Costa et al. (1988) used $^{99m}$Tc-HMPAO SPET in a study which included the scanning of Parkinson's disease patients during an 'on' phase of treatment with L-dopa and also during an 'off' phase after withdrawal of treatment. Using this paradigm, changes in blood flow in caudate and thalamus could be detected between the two states. Parkinson's disease offers many other exciting possibilities for study with neuroactivation. Some patients develop on/off fluctuations where they are doing well clinically and then suddenly 'freeze' and become rigid. SPET scanning during these two different states, especially using dopamine-specific ligands, would be quite revealing of the underlying neurotransmitter changes in this disease.

## Alzheimer's Disease

One of the richest potential areas for SPET neuroactivation is the field of geriatrics and the study of dementias. Using SPET, some researchers have investigated the effect on Alzheimer's disease patients of administration of drugs acting on the cholinergic system, thought to be deficient in AD (Battisstin et al. 1989). These studies have shown rCBF enhancement in the affected regions of AD with the drugs.

Clinically, frontal activation tasks might be used to judge response to treatment for a depressive pseudodementia patient. An example of this line of approach is shown in Fig. 2. A geriatric patient with depression is scanned first under a control situation and, for the second scan, is asked to generate new words for 2 min, each beginning with the letters 'F', 'A', 'S' similar to the protocol described in Chap. 9. Regional variations in response to activation protocols such as this may prove of benefit in earlier diagnoses, in dictating treatment and in evaluating response to therapy of patients with dementia.

# Future Applications

The potential clinical and research uses of SPET neuroactivation are vast. We have seen how this technique is already being used by some researchers to study the brain in various disease states. Below we review some of these new potentials.

## Earlier and More Accurate Diagnosis of Disease

PET has been shown to be more sensitive than MRI or a trained clinician in pre-morbid prediction of who will later develop Huntington's disease from among at-risk individuals. SPET is also sensitive to these pre-morbid changes in

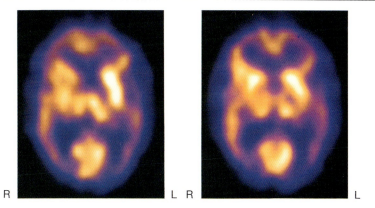

Fig 2. HMPAO SPET scans of a geriatric patient with depression (pseudodementia) during a control (*left*) and task (*right*). Note the activation of the frontal lobes, which may help distinguish these patients from those afflicted with a frontal dementia such as Pick's disease and help guide clinicians to aggressive use of antidepressant treatments (Chap. 9). (We gratefully acknowledge Dr. Michael Philpot for the use of this case.)

Huntington's disease. Theoretically, by using an activation task that dissects out the fundamental pathology of the disease, or that highlights the affected neuroanatomic systems, SPET could be made even more sensitive. This might make pre-morbid diagnosis of at-risk individuals easier.

The same principle, developing a SPET neuroactivation protocol that examined particular brain functions, could theoretically improve pre-morbid diagnosis in several neuropsychiatric disorders. As an example, suppose that a protective medication were found to delay effectively the progression of Parkinson's disease. A sensitive SPET neuroactivation task that examined the basal ganglia might allow for accurate diagnosis and treatment of PD at the first sign of a slight symptom such as axial rigidity or a mild tremor. Accurate diagnosis at an early stage would be even more important if the treatment were extremely costly or had other associated morbidity. The same possibility exists with Huntington's disease and schizophrenia. First-degree relatives that are at risk of developing the disorder could conceivably have a neuroactivated SPET scan that highlighted the appropriate neuroanatomic pathways and aided in pre-morbid diagnosis. Unfortunately, many of these neuroactivation studies in specific diseases must first wait for the development of reliable and appropriate activation protocols and normative data. However, SPET neuroactivation as an aid to diagnosis of many neuropsychiatric diseases is not far away.

## Predicting Response to Treatment

SPET neuroactivation may prove helpful in evaluating many neuropsychiatric treatments that directly affect brain function. At present, when most treatments in neurology and psychiatry are administered evaluation of the response must wait for weeks or months. SPET neuroactivation offers the promise of shortening the time to evaluate response by directly imaging brain function. This is particularly exciting in the area of stroke research. SPET can directly image blood flow to ischaemic areas. SPET scans before and after a vasodilating or anti-ischaemic agent could allow for quick evaluation and possible titration of the therapy. Again, in stroke management, often the brain recovers a function that was lost in a CVA. We currently know very little about the processes the brain uses to recover these lost functions, even when there has been extensive damage. SPET offers the possibility of revealing the 'alternative recruitment' methods used by the brain. Conceivably, by better understanding this process, we might be able to reformulate and improve our physical rehabilitation treatment methods.

## Understanding Disease Mechanisms

Finally, SPET neuroactivation is already allowing us better understanding of the fundamental mechanisms of neuropsychiatric disease processes. SPET can study the progressive changes in blood flow, so important to understanding cerebrovascular disease. However, in addition to studying simple blood flow SPET can study fundamental neurochemistry over time. When coupled with specific ligands, SPET allows us to understand the fundamental neurobiology and neurochemistry of diseases.

Thus, SPET neuroactivation has a vast potential for evaluating different treatment methods. The potential applications, clinically and in research, in health and in disease, for SPET and neuroactivation are limited only by our own energies and the ability to think of new ways of applying this exciting new technology.

# References

Bajc M, Medved V, Basic M, et al (1989) Acute effect of electroconvulsive therapy on brain perfusion assessed by Tc99m-hexamethylpropylene-amine oxime and single proton emission tomography. Acta Psychiatr Scand 80:421–426

Battisstin L, Pizzolato G, Dam M, et al (1989) Single-photon emission computed tomography studies with 99m-Tc-hexamethylpropyleneamine oxime in dementia: effects of acute administration of L-acetylcarnitine. Eur Neurol 29:261–265

Biersack HJ, Linke D, Brassel F, et al (1987) Technetium-99m HMPAO brain SPECT in epileptic patients before and during unilateral hemispheric anesthesia (Wada test): report of three cases. J Nucl Med 28:1763–1767

Chollet F, Celsis P, Clanet M, et al (1989) SPECT study of cerebral blood flow reactivity after acetazolamide in patients with transient ischaemic attacks. Stroke 20:458–464

Delecluse F, Voordecker P, Raftopoulos C (1989) Vertebrobasilar insufficiency revealed by xenon-133 inhalation SPECT. Stroke 20:952–956

Homan RW, Paulman RG, Devous MD, et al (1989) Cognitive function and regional cerebral blood flow in partial seizures. Arch Neurol 46:964–970

Hunter R, McLuskie R, Wyper D, et al (1989) The pattern of function-related regional cerebral blood flow investigated by single photon emission tomography with 99mTc-HMPAO in patients with presenile Alzheimer's disease and Korsakoff's psychosis. Psychol Med 19:847–855

Lang W, Podreka I, Suess E, et al (1988) Single photon emission computerized tomography during and between seizures. J Neurol 235:277–284

Matsuda H, Higashi S, Asli IN, et al (1988) Evaluation of cerebral collateral circulation by technetium-99m HMPAO brain SPECT during Matas test: report of three cases. J Nucl Med 29:1724–1729

Musalek M, Podreka I, Suess E, et al (1988) Neurophysiological aspects of auditory hallucinations. $^{99m}$Tc-(HMPAO)–SPECT investigations in patients with auditory hallucinations and normal controls – a preliminary report. Psychopathology 21:275–280

Notardonato H, Gonzales-Avilez A, Van Heertum RL, et al (1989) The potential value of serial cerebral SPECT scanning in the evaluation of psychiatric illness. Clin Nucl Med 14:319–322

Pilowski L, Costa DC, Kerwin R, et al (1991) Central D-2 dopaminergic receptor studies in treatment responsive and treatment resistant schizophrenia patients as measured by $^{123}$I-IBZM SPET (abstract). Schiz Res (in press)

Volkow ND, Wolf AP, Van Gelder P, et al (1987) Phenomenological correlates of metabolic activity in 18 patients with chronic schizophrenia. Am J Psychiatry 144:151–158

# Appendixes

## Appendix I

### Area-Specific Activation Tasks

| Brain area to investigate | Test or task | Established and confirmed?[a] |
|---|---|---|
| **Cognitive or motor tasks** | | |
| Frontal lobes | Stroop Color Chart | PET, EP |
| | Wisconsin Card Sort | PET, EP |
| Parietal lobe | | |
|   Motor strip | Moving contralateral limb | PET, EP |
|   Right side | Spatial image processing | PET, EP |
| Cerebellum | Moving ipsilateral limb | PET, EP |
| Temporal lobes | | |
|   left | Speaking, listening | PET, EP, SPET |
| | Silent answering of language | |
| Occipital lobes | Visual imagery | PET, EP, SPET |
| | Strobing light | |
| **Pharmacological** | | |
| Parietal lobes (Cholinergic system) | L-Acetyl carnitine | SPET |
| Middle cerebral artery diameter (vasoreactivity) | Nitroglycerin | SPET |
| | Acetazolamide | |

[a] PET, Proven by pet scanning; EP, demonstrated electrophysiologically; SPET, demonstrated by SPET scanning. For the tasks not yet proven by SPET, one

cannot conclude that a failure to activate this brain region on a SPET study means the patient has pathology. As explained in the text, technological and methodological differences may allow an area to be demonstrably activated by PET and not by SPET and vice versa.

# Appendix II

## A Guide to Performing Neuroactivation Studies

1 Choose the brain region or function that you wish to investigate.

    Relevant issues: Does the area covary with other brain regions, or is it relatively independent?

2 Choose the appropriate active versus control task or pharmacological probe for that area (from Appendix I).

    Relevant issues:
- Is the task reproducible?
- Can it be maintained for the necessary amount of time for tracer deposition?
- Has it been shown by others to activate the appropriate brain areas?
- Does the control task isolate the active function and not involve other variables?

3 Choose the radionuclide tracer and scanning instrument.
(See discussion in Chaps. 2 and 3)

    Relevant issues: $^{99m}$Tc-HMPAO
$^{123}$IMP
$^{133}$X

- Does the chosen tracer have the appropriate half-life and deposition time for the task?
- How much resolution can the instrument provide?

4 Depending on the uptake kinetics and half-life of the tracer, decide on the activation and control protocol.

    Relevant issues:
- Task and control on the same day or return in several weeks?

5 Choose the appropriate data analysis method.

    Relevant issues: Region of interest or covariant analysis?

# Selected Bibliography

See also specific references at the end of each chapter

Abdel-Dayem HM, Bahar RK, Sigurdsson GH, et al (1989) The hollow skull: a sign of brain death in Tc-99m HM-PAO brain scintigraphy. Clin Nucl Med 14:912–916
Ackerman RH (1984) On cerebral blood flow, stroke and SPECT. Stroke 15:1–4
Adams RD, Victor M (1989) Principles of neurology, 4th edn. McGraw Hill, New York
Alexander GE, De Long MR, Strick PL (1986) Parallel organization of functionally segregated circuits linking basal ganglia and cortex. Ann Rev Neurosci 9:357–381
Andersen AR, Friberg HH, Schmidt JF, et al (1988) Quantitative measurements of cerebral blood flow using SPECT and 99mTc-d, l-HM-PAO compared to xenon-133. J Cereb Blood Flow Metab 8:S69–S81
Anderson AR, Friberg H, Knudsen K, et al (1988) Extraction of 99mTc-d-l-HMPAO across the blood brain barrier. J Cereb Blood Flow Metab 8:544–551
Anderson AR, Friberg L, Olsen TS, et al (1988) SPECT demonstration of delayed hyperemia following hypoperfusion in classic migraine. Arch Neurol 45:154–159
Andreasen NC (1988) Evaluation of brain imaging techniques in mental illness. Ann Rev Med 39:335–345
Ashwal S, Schneider S, Thompson J (1989) Xenon computed tomography measuring cerebral blood flow in the determination of brain death in children. Ann Neurol 25:539–546
Bajc M, Medved V, Basic M, et al (1989) Acute effect of electroconvulsive therapy on brain perfusion assessed by Tc99m-hexamethylpropylene-amineoxime and single photon emission tomography. Acta Psychiat Scand 80:421–426
Batjer HH, Devous MD, Meyer MJ, et al (1988) Cerebrovascular haemodynamics in arteriovenous malformation complicated by normal perfusion pressure breakthrough. Neurosurgery 22:503–509
Battisstin L, Pizzolato G, Dam M, et al (1989) Single-photon emission computed tomography studies with 99m-Tc-hexamethylpropyleneamine oxime in dementia: effects of acute administration of L-acetylcarnitine. Eur Neurol 29:261–265
Battistella PA, Ruffilli R, Pozza FD, et al (1990) 99Tc HM-PAO SPECT in pediatric migraine. Headache 30:646–649
Bauer J, Stefan H, Huk WJ, et al (1989) CT, MRI and SPECT neuroimaging in status epilepticus with simple partial and complex partial seizures: case report. J Neurol 236:296–299
Baxter LR (1990) Brain imaging as a tool in establishing a theory of brain pathology in obsessive compulsive disorder. J Clin Psychiatry 51:S22–S25
Baxter LR, Phelps ME, Mazziota JC, et al (1987) Local cerebral glucose metabolic rates in obsessive-compulsive disorder. Arch Gen Psychiatry 44:211–218
Baxter LR, Schwartz JM, Mazziotta JC, et al (1988) Cerebral glucose metabolic rates in non-depressed patients with obsessive-compulsive disorder. Am J Psychiatry 145:1560–1563
Beer HF, Blauenstein PA, Hasler PH, et al (1990) In vitro and in vivo evaluation of iodine-123-Ro-16-0154: a new imaging agent for SPECT investigations of benzodiazepine receptors. J Nucl Med 31:1007–1014
Biersack HJ, Linke D, Brassel F, et al (1987) Technetium-99m HM-PAO brain SPECT in epileptic patients before and during unilateral hemispheric anesthesia (Wada test): report of three cases. J Nucl Med 28:1763–1767

Brott TG, Gelfand MJ, Williams CC, et al (1986) Frequency and patterns of abnormality detected by iodine-123 amine emission CT after cerebral infarction. Radiology 158:729–734

Burns A, Philpot MP, Costa DC, et al (1989) The investigation of Alzheimer's disease with single photon emission tomography. J Neurol Neurosurg Psychiatry 52:248–253

Chiron C, Raynaud C, Tzourio N, et al (1989) Regional cerebral blood flow by SPECT imaging in Sturge-Weber disease: an aid for diagnosis. J Neurol Neurosurg Psychiatry 52:1402–1409

Chollet F, Celsis P, Clanet M (1989) SPECT study of cerebral blood flow reactivity after acetazolamide in patients with transient ischaemic attacks. Stroke 20:458–464

Churchland PM (1984) Matter and consciousness. MIT Press, Cambridge

Churchland PM (1988) Neurophilosophy: toward a unified science of the mind-brain. MIT Press, Cambridge

Churchland PM (1989) A neurocomputational perspective. MIT Press, Cambridge, pp 153–230

Clark CM, Kessler R, Margolin R (1985) The statistical interaction of cerebral specialization and integration in the interpretation of dynamic brain images. Brain Cogn 4:7–12

Cohen MB, Lake RR, Graham LS, et al (1989) Quantitative iodine-123 IMP imaging of brain perfusion in schizophrenia. J Nucl Med 30:1616–1620

Costa DC, Ell PJ, Cullum ID, et al (1986) The in vivo distribution of $^{99}Tc^m$-HM-PAO in normal man. Nuclear Med Commun 7:647–658

Costa DC, Ell PJ, Burns A, et al (1988) CBF tomograms and Tc-HM-PAO in patients with dementia (Alzheimer's type and HIV) and Parkinson's disease – initial results. J Cereb Blood Flow Metab 8:S109–S115

Crick F (1989) The recent excitement about neural networks. Nature 337:129–132

Dahl A, Russel D, Nyberg-Hansen R, et al (1989) Effect of nitroglycerin on cerebral circulation measured by transcranial Doppler and SPECT. Stroke 20:1733–1736

Damasio H, Damasio AR (1989) Lesion analysis in neuropsychology. Oxford University Press, New York

Defer G, Moretti JL, Cesaro P, et al (1987) Early and delayed SPECT using N-isopropyl prognostic index for clinical recovery. Arch Neurol 44:715–718

Delecluse F, Voordecker P, Raftopoulos C (1989) Vertebrobasilar insufficiency revealed by xenon-133 inhalation SPECT. Stroke 20:952–956

Denays R, Tondeur M, Foulon M, et al (1989) Regional brain blood flow in congenital dysphasia: studies with technetium-99m-HMPAO SPECT. J Nucl Med 30:1825–1829

Denays R, Tondeur M, Toppet V, et al (1990) Cerebral palsy: initial experience with Tc-99m HMPAO SPECT of the brain. Radiology 175:111–116

Descartes R (1987) Meditation II. In: Haldane ES, Ross GRT (trans) The philosophical works of Descartes. Cambridge University Press, Cambridge

Duncan R, Patterson J, Hadley DM, Macpherson P, Brodie MJ, Bone I, McGeorge AP, Wyper DJ (1990) CT, MR and SPECT imaging in temporal lobe epilepsy. J Neurol Neurosurg Psychiatry 53:11–15

Ell PJ (1990) Single photon emission computed tomography (SPET) of the brain. J Neurosci Meth 34:207–217

Ell PJ, Williams ES (1981) Nuclear medicine: an introductory text. Blackwell Scientific, London

Ell PJ, Cullum I, Costa DC (1885) Regional cerebral blood flow mapping with a new Tc-99m-labelled compound. Lancet I:50–51

Ell PJ, Hocknell JML, Jarritt P (1985) A $^{99}Tc^m$-labelled radiotracer for the investigation of cerebral vascular disease. Nucl Med Commun 6:437–441

Ell PJ, Costa DC, Cullum ID, et al (1987) The clinical application of rCBF imaging by SPET. Amersham International, Little Chalfont, England

Ell PJ, Jarritt PH, Costa DC, et al (1987) Functional imaging of the brain. Semin Nucl Med 17:214–229

Engel J (1984) The use of positron emission tomographic scanning in epilepsy. Ann Neurol 15:S180–S191

Evans DW, Hill DJ (1987) Brain death. Lancet I:102–102

Fish DR, Brooks DJ, Young IR, Bydder GM (1988) Use of magnetic resonance imaging to identify changes in cerebral blood flow in epilepsia partialis continua. Magn Reson Med 8:238–240

Fogel B (1990) Localization in neuropsychiatry. J Neuropsychiatry 2:361–362

Fox PT (1989) Functional brain mapping with positron emission tomography. Sem Neurol 9:323–329

Fox PT, Perlmutter SS, Raichle ME (1988) Enhanced detection of focal brain enzymes using intersubject averaging and change-distribution analysis of subtracted PET images. J Cereb Blood Flow Metab 8:642–653

Friston KJ, Passingham RE, Nutt JG, et al (1989) Localization in PET images: direct fitting of the intercommissural (AC-PC) line. J Cereb Blood Flow Metab 9:690–695

Galaske RG, Schober O, Heyer R (1988) $^{99m}$Tc-HM-PAO and $^{123}$I-amphetamine cerebral scintigraphy: a new, non-invasive method in determination of brain death in children. Eur J Nucl Med 14:446–452

Galaske RG, Schober O, Heyer R (1989) Determination of brain death in children with $^{123}$I-IMP and Tc-99m HMPAO. Psychiatry Res 29:343–345

Gemmell HG, Sharp PF, Besson JA, et al (1987) Differential diagnosis in dementia using the cerebral blood flow agent $^{99m}$Tc HM-PAO: a SPECT study. J Comput Assist Tomogr 11:398–402

George MS (1987) Neuroscience and Psychiatry. Am J Psychiatry 144:1103

George MS (1990) Establishing brain death: the potential role of nuclear medicine in the search for a reliable confirmatory test. Eur J Nucl Med 18:75–77

George MS, Robertson MM, Costa DC, et al (1991) HMPAO SPECT Scans of co-morbid OCD/GTS patients. APA Symposium Abstracts: (Abstract)

George MS, Robertson MM, Costa DC, et al (1991) D2 receptor activity in Tourette syndrome (GTS). APA Symposium Abstracts: (Abstract)

George MS, Costa DC, Kouris K, et al (1991) $^{99}$Tc$^m$-HMPAO abnormalities in infantile autism. APA (Abstract)

George MS, Ring HA, Costa DC, et al (1991) Demonstration of human parietal lobe activation using SPET (abstract). Nucl Med Commun 12:273

Geschwind N (1965) Disconnexion syndromes in animals and man. Brain 88:585–644

Geschwind N (1965) Disconnexion syndromes in animals and man. Brain 88:237–294

Gilman S, Adams K, Koeppe RA, et al (1990) Cerebellar and frontal hypometabolism in alcoholic cerebellar degeneration studied with PET. Ann Neurol 28:775–785

Ginsberg MD, Yoshii F, Vibulsresth S, et al (1987) Human task-specific somatosensory activation. Neurology 37:1301–1308

Goldenberg G, Podreka I, Steiner M, et al (1987) Patterns of regional cerebral blood flow related to memorizing of high and low imagery words – an emission computer tomography study. Neuropsychologia 25:473–485

Goldenberg G, Podreka I, Uhl F, et al (1989) Cerebral correlates of imagining colours, faces and a map. I.SPECT of regional cerebral blood flow. Neuropsychologia 27:1315–1328

Goldenberg G, Podreka I, Steiner M, et al (1989) Regional cerebral blood flow patterns in visual imagery. Neuropsychologia 27:641–664

Greenberg JH, Kushner M, Rango M, et al (1990) Validation studies of iodine-123-iodoamphetamine as a cerebral blood flow tracer using emission tomography. J Nucl Med 31:1364–1369

Gur RC, Trivedi SS, Saykin AJ, et al (1988) Behavioral imaging: a procedure for the analysis and display of neuropsychological test scores. I. Construction of the algorithm and initial clinical evaluation. Neuropsychiatr Neuropsychol Behav Neural 1:53–60

Gur RE, Gur RC, Skolnick BE, et al (1985) Brain function in psychiatric disorders. III. Regional cerebral blood flow in unmedicated schizophrenics. Arch Gen Psychol 42:329–334

Hamlin CL, Swayne LC, Liebowitz MR (1989) Striatal IMP-SPECT decrease in obsessive-compulsive disorder, normalized by pharmacotherapy. Neuropsychia Neuropsychol Behav Neural 2:290–300

Hawton K, Shepstone B, Soper N, et al (1990) Single-photon emission computerized tomography (SPECT) in schizophrenia. Br J Psychiatry 156:425–427

Hill EG, George MS (1987) Sir Thomas Willis and the seventeenth century understanding of headache. Neurology (abstract)

Hill TC, Holman BL, Lovett R, et al (1982) Initial experience with SPECT of the brain using N-isopropyl-(I-123)-p-iodoamphetamine. J Nucl Med 23:191–195

Hill TC, Magistretti PL, Holman BL, et al (1984) Assessment of regional cerebral blood flow (rCBF) in stroke using SPECT and N-isopropyl-(I-123)-p-iodoamphetamine. Stroke 15:40–45

Holman BL (1986) Perfusion and receptor SPECT in the dementias. J Nucl Med 27:855–860

Holman BL, Tumeh SS (1990) Single-photon emission computed tomography (SPECT). JAMA 263:561–564

Holman BL, Hellman RS, Goldsmith SJ, et al (1989) Biodistribution, dosimetry and clinical evaluation of Tc-99m ethyl cysteinate dimer (ECD) in normal subjects and in patients with chronic cerebral infarction. J Nucl Med 30:1018–1024

Homan RW, Paulman RG, Devous MD, et al (1989) Cognitive function and regional cerebral blood flow in partial seizures. Arch Neurol 46:964–970

Hunter R, McLuskie R, Wyper D, et al (1989) The pattern of function-related regional cerebral blood flow investigated by single photon emission tomography with $^{99m}$Tc-HMPAO in patients with presenile Alzheimer's disease and Korsakoff's psychosis. Psychol Med 19:847–855

Johnson KA, Holman BL, Rosen TJ, et al (1991) I-123 IMP SPECT is accurate in the diagnosis of Alzheimer's disease. Arch Intern Med (in press)

Kandel ER, Schwartz JH (1981) Principles of neural science. Elsevier/North Holland, New York, pp 324

Katz A, Bose A, Lind SJ, et al (1990) SPECT in patients with epilepsia partialis continua. Neurology 40:1848–1850

Kelly PAT, Faulkner AJ, Burrow AP (1989) The effects of the GABA agonist muscimol upon blood flow in different vascular territories of the rat cortex. J Cereb Blood Flow Metab 9:754–758

Kim CK, Palestro CJ, Goldsmith SJ (1990) SPECT imaging in the diagnosis of Budd-Chiari syndrome. J Nucl Med 31:109–111

Kim KT, Black KL, Marciano D, et al (1990) Thallium-201 SPECT imaging of brain tumors: methods and results. J Nucl Med 31:965–969

Korein J, Braunstein P, George A (1977) Brain death I: angiographic correlation of the radioisotope bolus technique for evaluation of critical deficit of cerebral blood flow. Ann Neurol 2:195–205

Kuhn TS (1962) The structure of scientific revolutions. University of Chicago Press, Chicago

Kung HF, Alavi A, Chang W, et al (1990) In vivo SPECT imaging of CNS D-2 dopamine receptors: initial studies with iodine-123-IBZM in humans. J Nucl Med 31:573–579

Kushner MJ, Tobin M, Fazekas F, et al (1990) Cerebral blood flow variations in CNS lupus. Neurology 40:99–102

Lammertsma AA, Frackowiak RSJ, Hoffman JM, et al (1989) The C1502 build-up technique to measure regional cerebral blood-flow and volume of distribution of water. J Cereb Blood Flow Metab 9:461–470

Lang W, Podreka I, Suess E, et al (1988) Single photon emission computerized tomography during and between seizures. J Neurol 235:277–284

Lang W, Lang M, Podreka I, et al (1988) DC-potential shifts and regional cerebral blood flow reveal frontal cortex involvement in human visuomotor learning. Exp Brain Res 71:353–364

Langen KJ, Coenen HH, Roosen N, et al (1990) SPECT studies of brain tumors with L-3-[123I] iodo-alpha-methyl tyrosine: comparison with PET, $^{124}$IMT and first clinical results. J Nucl Med 31:281–286

Lashley KS (1937) Functional determinants of cerebral localization. Arch Neurol Psychiatry 38:371–387

Lassen NA, Roland PE, Larsen B, et al (1977) Mapping of human cerebral functions: a study of the regional cerebral blood flow pattern during rest, its reproducibility and the activations seen during basic sensory and motor functions. Acta Neurol Scand 56 [Suppl 64]:262–263

Lassen NA, Ingvar DH, Skinhoj E (1978) Brain function and blood flow. Sci Am 239:62–71

Lassen NA, Andersen AR, Friberg L, et al (1988) The retention of [$^{99m}$Tc]-d,l-HM-PAO in the human brain after intracarotid bolus injection: kinetic analysis. J Cereb Blood Flow Metab 8[Suppl 1]:S13–S22

Lauritzen M, Olsen TS, Lassen NA, et al (1983) Changes in regional cerebral blood flow during the course of classic migraine attacks. Ann Neurol 13:633–641

Lee BI, Markand ON, Wellman HN, et al (1987) HIPDM single photon emission computed tomography brain imaging in partial onset secondarily generalized tonic clonic seizures. Epilepsia 28:305–311

Lee BI, Markand ON, Wellman HN, et al (1988) HIPDM-SPECT in patients with medically intractable complex partial seizures: ictal study. Arch Neurol 45:397–402

Lehky SR, Sejnowski TR (1988) Network model of shape-from-shading: neural function arises from both receptive and projective fields. Nature 333:452–454

Levine SR, Welch KMA, Ewing JR, et al (1987) Asymmetric cerebral blood flow patterns in migraine. Cephalalgia 7:245–248

Lim CB, Walker R, Pinkstaff C, et al (1986) Triangular SPECT system for 3-D total organ volume imaging: performance, results and dynamic imaging quality. IEEE Trans Nucl Sci 33:501–504

Linsker R (1986) From basic network principles to neural architecture: emergence of orientation columns. Proc Natl Acad Sci 83:8779–8783

Lou HC, Henriksen L, Bruhn P (1990) Focal cerebral dysfunction in developmental learning disabilities. Lancet 335:8–11

Luria AR (1980) Higher cortical functions in man, 2nd edn. Basic Books, New York

Malsburg C von der, Singer W (1988) Principles of cortical network organization. In: Rakic P, Singer W (eds) Neurobiology of neocortex. John Wiley, Chichester, pp 69–99

Matsuda H, Higashi S, Asli IN, et al (1988) Evaluation of cerebral collateral circulation by

technetium-99m HM-PAO brain SPECT during Matas test: report of three cases. J Nucl Med 29:1724–1729
Maurer AH, Siegel JA, Comerota AJ, et al (1990) SPECT quantification of cerebral ischemia before and after carotid endarterectomy. J Nucl Med 31:1412–1420
Mazziotta JC, Phelps ME (1984) Human sensory stimulation and deprivation: positron emission tomographic results and strategies. Ann Neurol 15:S50–S60
Mazziotta JC, Phelps ME (1986) Positron emission tomography studies of the brain. In: Phelps M, Mazziotta J, Schelbert H (eds) Positron emission tomography and autoradiography: principles and applications for the brain and heart. Raven Press, New York, pp 493–579
McClelland JL, Rumelhart DE, The PDP research group (1986) Parallel distributed processing, vol 2. MIT Press, Cambridge, Massachusetts
Mesulam MM (1985) Principles of behavioral neurology. Davis, Philadelphia
Mesulam MM (1990) Large-scale neurocognitive networks and distributed processing for attention, language and memory. Ann Neurol 28:597–613
Mettler EJ, Riege WH, Kuhl DE, et al (1984) Cerebral metabolic relationships for selected brain regions in healthy adults. J Cereb Blood Flow Metab 4:1–7
Metter EJ, Hanson WR, Jackson CA, et al (1990) Temporoparietal cortex in aphasia: evidence from PET. Arch Neurol 47:1235–1238
Mintun MA, Fox PT, Raichle ME (1989) A highly accurate method of localizing regions of neuronal activation in the human brain with positron emission tomography. J Cereb Blood Flow Metab 9:96–103
Montaldi D, Brooks DN, McColl JH, et al (1990) Measurements of regional cerebral blood flow and cognitive performance in Alzheimer's disease. J Neurol Neurosurg Psychiat 53:33–38
Mountz JM, Modell JG, Foster NL, et al (1990) Prognostication of recovery following stroke using the comparison of CT and technetium-99m HM-PAO SPECT. J Nucl Med 31:61–66
Musalek M, Podreka I, Walter H, et al (1987) Regional brain function in hallucinations: a study of regional cerebral blood flow in 99m-Tc-HM-PAO SPECT in patients with auditory hallucinations, tactile hallucinations and normal controls. Compr Psychiatry 30:89–108
Musalek M, Podreka I, Suess E, et al (1988) Neurophysiological aspects of auditory hallucinations. $^{99m}$Tc-(HMPAO) – SPECT investigations in patients with auditory hallucinations and normal controls – a preliminary report. Psychopathology 21:275–280
Nagel JS, Johnson KA, Ichise M, et al (1988) Decreased iodine-123 IMP caudate nucleus uptake in patients with Huntington's disease. Clin Nucl Med 13:486–490
Neary D, Snowden JS, Mann DMA, et al (1990) Frontal lobe dementia and motor neuron disease. J Neurol Neurosurg Psychiatry 53:23–32
Nelson ME, Bower JM (1990) Brain maps and parallel computers. Trends Neurosci 13:403–408
Nordahl TE, Benkelfat C, Semple WE, et al (1989) Cerebral glucose metabolic rates in obsessive-compulsive disorder. Neuropsychopharmacology 2:23–28
Notardonato H, Gonzales-Avilez A, Van Heertum RL, et al (1989) The potential value of serial cerebral SPECT scanning in the evaluation of psychiatric illness. Clin Nucl Med 14:319–322
O'Connell RA, Van Heertum RL, Billick SB, et al (1989) Single photon emission computed tomography (SPECT) with IMP in the differential diagnosis of psychiatric disorders. J Neuropsychiatry 1:145–153
Oleson J, Larsen B, Lauritzen M (1981) Focal hyperemia followed by spreading oligemia and impaired activation of rCBF in classic migraine. Ann Neurol 9:344–352
Pardo JV, Pardo PJ, Janer KW, et al (1990) The anterior cingulate cortex mediates processing selection in the Stroop attentional conflict paradigm. Neurobiology 87:256–259
Paulman RG, Devous MD, Gregory RR, et al (1990) Hypofrontality and cognitive impairment in schizophrenia: dynamic single-photon tomography and neuropsychological assessment of schizophrenic brain function. Biol Psychiatry 27:377–399
Penfield W, Rasmussen T (1950) The cerebral cortex of man. Macmillan, New York
Petersen SE, Fox PT, Posner MI, et al (1988) Positron emission tomographic studies of the cortical anatomy of single-word processing. Nature 331:585–589
Pilowski L, Costa DC, Kerwin R, et al (1991) Central D-2 dopaminergic receptor studies in treatment responsive and treatment resistant schizophrenia patients as measured by 123 I-IBZM SPET. Schiz Res 4:410
Podreka I, Suess E, Goldenberg G, et al. (1987) Initial experience with technetium-99m-HM-PAO brain SPECT. J Nucl Med 28:1657–1666
Prohovnik I, Hakansson K, Risberg J (1980) Observations on the functional significance of regional cerebral blood flow in "resting" normal subjects. Neuropsychologia 18:203–217
Raichle ME (1987) Circulatory and metabolic correlates of brain function. In: Plum F (ed) The

nervous system: higher functions of the brain. American Physiological Society, Bethesda, pp 643–674
Rango M, Candelise L, Perani D, et al (1989) Cortical pathophysiology and clinical neurologic abnormalities in acute cerebral ischemia. A serial study with single photon emission computed tomography. Arch Neurol 46:1318–1322
Reed BR, Jagust WJ, Seab JP, et al (1989) Memory and regional cerebral blood flow in mildly symptomatic Alzheimer's disease. Neurology 39:1537–1539
Reid RH, Gulenchyn KY, Ballinger JR (1989) Clinical use of technetium-99m HM-PAO for determination of brain death. J Nucl Med 30:1621–1626
Reid RH, Gulenchyn KY, Ballinger JR, et al (1990) Cerebral perfusion imaging with technetium-99m HMPAO following cerebral trauma. Clin Nucl Med 15:383–388
Ring HA, George MS, Costa DC, et al (1991) The use of cerebral activation procedures with single photon emission tomography (SPET): a review. Eur J Nucl Med 18:133–141
Risberg J (1987) Development of high-resolution two-dimensional measurement of regional cerebral blood flow. In: Wade J, Knezevic S, Maximilian VA, Mubrin Z, Prohvnic I (eds) Impact of functional imaging in neurology and psychiatry. Libbey, London, pp 35–43
Risberg J (1989) Regional cerebral blood flow measurements with high temporal and spatial resolution. In: Ottson D, Rostene W (eds) Visulization of brain functions. Wenner-Gren International Symposium Series, vol 53. Macmillan Press, London, pp 153–158
Roine RO, Launes J, Lindroth L, Nikkinen P (1986) $^{99m}$Tc-Hexamethylpropyleneamine oxime scans to confirm brain death. Lancet II: 1223–1224
Roland PE, Friberg L (1985) Localization of cortical areas activated by thinking. J Neurophysiol 53:1219–1243
Rorty R (1971) In defense of eliminative materialism. In: Rosenthal DM (ed) Materialism and the mind-body problem. Prentice-Hall, Englewood Cliffs
Rowe CC, Berkovic SS, Austin M, et al (1984) Postictal SPET in epilepsy. Lancet I:389–390
Rubinstein M, Denays R, Ham HR, et al (1989) Functional imaging of brain maturation in humans using iodine-123-iodoamphetamine and SPECT. J Nucl Med 30:1982–1985
Rumelhart DE, McClelland JL, The PDP Research Group (1986) Parallel distributed processing, vol 1. MIT Press, Cambridge
Rumsey JM, Duara R, Grady C, et al (1985) Brain metabolism in autism. Resting cerebral glucose utilization rates as measured with positron emission tomography. Arch Gen Psychiatry 42:448–455
Ryding E, Rosen I, Elmqvist D, et al (1988) SPECT measurements with $^{99}$Tc-HM-PAO in focal epilepsy. J Cereb Blood Flow Metab 8:595–601
Ryle G (1949) The concept of mind. Hutchinson, London
Sakai F, Meyer JS, Naritomi H, et al (1978) Regional cerebral blood flow and EEG in patients with epilepsy. Arch Neurol 35:648–657
Schlake HP, Bottger IG, Grotemeyer KH, et al (1989) Brain imaging with $^{123}$I-IMP SPECT in migraine between attacks. Headache 29:344–349
Schwartz JM, Baxter LR, Mazziotta JC, et al (1987) The differential diagnosis of depression: relevance of positron emission tomography studies of cerebral glucose metabolism to the bipolar-unipolar dichotomy. JAMA 258:1368–1374
Schwartz JM, Speed NM, Mountz JM, et al (1990) $^{99m}$Tc-Hexamethylpropyleneamine oxime single photon emission CT in poststroke depression. Am J Psychiatry 147:242–244
Seibyl JP, Krystal JH, Goodman WK, Price LH (1989) Obsessive-compulsive symptoms in a patient with a right frontal lobe lesion. Neuropsychia Neuropsychol Behav Neurol 1:295–299
Seiderer M, Krappel W, Moser E, et al (1989) Detection and quantification of chronic cerebrovascular disease: comparison of MR imaging, SPECT and CT. Radiology 170:545–548
Shahar E, Gilday DL, Hwang PA, et al (1990) Pediatric cerebrovascular disease: alterations of regional cerebral blood flow detected by Tc-99m-HMPAO SPECT. Arch Neurol 47:578–584
Sharp PF, Smith FW, Gemmell HG, et al (1986) Technetium-99m-Tc-HM-PAO stereoisomers as potential agents for imaging regional cerebral blood flow. J Nucl Med 27:171–177
Shen W, Lee BI, Park HM, et al (1990) HIPDM-SPECT brain imaging in the presurgical evaluation of patients with intractable seizures. J Nucl Med 31:1280–1284
Sherman M, Nass R, Shapiro T (1984) Regional cerebral blood flow in infantile autism. J Autism Dev Dis 4:438–440
Smith DF, Smith FW, Knight RS, et al (1989) 99Tcm-HMPAO single photon emission computed tomography in partial epilepsy: a preliminary report. Br J Radiol 62:970–973
Smith FW, Besson JAO, Gemmell HG, et al (1988) The use of technetium-99m-HM-PAO in the

assessment of patients with dementia and other neuropsychiatric conditions. J Cereb Blood Flow Metab 8[Suppl 1]:S116–S122

Smythies JR, Beloff J (1989) The case for dualism. University Press of Virginia, Charlottesville

Sokoloff L (1977) Relation between physiological function and energy metabolism in the central nervous system. J Neurochem 29:13–26

Sokoloff L (1978) Local cerebral energy metabolism: its relationships to local functional activity and blood flow. In: Purves MJ, Elliott L (eds) Cerebral vascular smooth muscle and its control. Elsevier, Amsterdam, pp 171–197

Stilhard G, Landis T, Schiess R, et al. (1990) Bitemporal hypoperfusion in transient global amnesia: 99m-Tc-HM-PAO SPECT and neuropsychological findings during and after an attack. J Neurol Neurosurg Psychiatry 53:339–342

Stroop JR (1935) Studies of interference in serial verbal reactions. J Exp Psychol 18:643–662

Strub RL, Black WF (1988) Neurobehavioral disorders: a clinical approach. Davis, Philadelphia

Stuss DT, Benson DF (1986) The frontal lobes. Raven Press, New York

Swedo SE, Schapiro MB, Grady CL, et al (1989) Cerebral glucose metabolism in childhood-onset obsessive compulsive disorder. Arch Gen Psychiatry 46:518–523

Takehara Y, Takahashi M, Isoda H, et al (1989) Scintigraphic evaluation of brain death with $^{99m}$Tc-d,l-hexamethyl-propyleneamine oxime (HMPAO). Radioisotopes 38:335–338

Talairach J, Szilka G (1967) Atlas of stereotaxic anatomy of the telencephalon. Masson & Cie, Paris

Taylor J (1958) Selected writings of John Hughlings Jackson. Basic Books, New York

Terry RD, Katzman R (1983) Senile dementia of the Alzheimer's type. Ann Neurol 14:497–506

Townsend CE, Costa DC, Jarritt PH, et al (1991) The evaluation of a new three detector gamma camera (IGE Neurocam) in a clinical environment. In: Nuclear medicine: the state of the art of nuclear medicine in Europe. Schattauer, Stuttgart, pp 11–13

Toyama H, Takeshita G, Takeuchi A, et al (1990) Cerebral hemodynamics in patients with chronic obstructive carotid disease by rCBF, rCBV, and rCBV/rCBF ratio using SPECT. J Nucl Med 31:55–60

Trimble MR (1988) Biological psychiatry. John Wiley, Chichester

Tumeh SS, Nagel JS, English RJ, et al (1990) Cerebral abnormalities in cocaine abusers: demonstration by SPECT perfusion scintigraphy. Radiology 176:821–824

Van Heertum RL, Tikofsky RS (1989) Advances in cerebral SPECT imaging: an atlas and guideline for practitioners. Trivirum, New York

Volkow ND, Wolf AP, Van Gelder P, et al (1987) Phenomenological correlates of metabolic activity in 18 patients with chronic schizophrenia. Am J Psychiatry 144:151–158

Volpe BT, Herscovitch P, Raichle ME, et al (1983) Cerebral blood flow and metabolism in human amnesia. J Cereb Blood Flow Metab 3:S5–S6

Walker-Batson D, Wendt JS, Devous MD, et al (1988) A long-term follow-up case study of crossed aphasia assessed by single-photon emission tomography (SPECT), language, and neuropsychological testing. Brain Lang 33:311–322

Weinberger DR, Berman KF, Zec Rf (1986) Physiologic dysfunction of dorsolateral prefrontal cortex in schizophrenia. Arch Gen Psychiatry 43:114–124

Wessely P, Suess E, Koch G, et al (1989) SPECT (99m)Tc-HMPAO finding in acute headache and during symptom-free interval. Cephalalgia 9:62–63

Woods SW, Hegeman IM, Zubal IG, et al (1991) Visual stimulation increases technetium-99m-HMPAO distribution in human visual cortex. J Nucl Med 32:210–215

Yamaguchi S, Kobayashi S, Murata A, et al (1987) Regional cerebral blood flow in post-stroke depressive disorder. J Cereb Blood Flow Metab 7:S218

Yeo RA, Turkheimer E, Bigler ED (1990) Neuropsychological methods of localizing brain dysfunction: clinical versus empirical approaches. Neuropsychia Neuropsychol Behav Neurol 3:290–303

Young JZ (1986) Philosophy and the brain. Oxford University Press, Oxford

Zipser D, Andersen RA (1988) A back-propagation programmed network that simulates response properties of a sub-set of posterior parietal neurones. Nature 331:676–684

# Subject Index

Acetazolamide 145, 175
L-acetylcarnitine 145
Acquisition angle 36
Activation protocols
  in normal subjects 157
  in specific disease states 173
  methods 157
  time course of 158
Activation tasks
  area specific 181
  frontal 162
  parietal 160
  visual 168
AIDS dementia 68–70
  case histories 68–9
  image acquisition parameters 66, 68
ALARA (as low as reasonably achievable)
  principle 8, 47
Alzheimer's disease 58–62, 145, 178
  case histories 58–62
  image acquisition parameters 58, 59, 61
  neuroSPET picture 62
  SPET findings 61
Amino acids 21
Anatomical site neural computation and
  behaviour 140
Anger gamma camera 4, 5, 39, 40
Angular sampling 34
Annular single-crystal brain camera
  (ASPECT) 45
Anxiety 167
Attention-deficit and hyperactivity disorder
  (ADHD) 73
Attenuation 35
Auditory hallucinations 175, 176
Autism, infantile. See Infantile autism

Back-projection angle 36
Basal ganglia 179
Benzodiazepine receptor system 21
Blood–brain barrier
  characteristics of 11–13
  imaging 11
  radiopharmaceuticals 13–14
  radiotracers 13
  structural components of 12
Blood flow changes 180
Bodily humors 123
Brain activity, associated with performance
  tasks 143
Brain damage, behavioural consequences of
  141
Brain function
  imaging 179
  normal 157
Brain function localization 123
  historical review 123
  philosophical review 127
  phrenological view of 127
  recent views of 135
Brain lesion localization 124
Brain perfusion, radiopharmaceuticals 14
Brain perfusion reserve 14
Brain processing models 133
  central features of 135
  parallel distributed processing 136
Bromine 77-methyl-spiperone 25

$^{11}$C-labelled amino acids 14
Calibration procedure 38
Carbon dioxide 145
Carotid artery occlusion 146, 175
Cartesian dualism 128, 129, 130
Caudate nuclei 176
CBPAO 19, 20
Central nervous system 11
Cerebral blood flow 14, 148
Cerebral blood flow, reactivity 145
Cerebral blood volume,
  radiopharmaceuticals 14
Cerebral cortex 133, 135, 149
Cerebral global and frontal metabolic rate
  176
Cerebral lesions 138
Cerebral localization. See Brain function
  localization
Cerebral processes, effects of pathological
  states 143

Cerebrovascular accidents 138
Cerebrovascular diseases 13, 18, 80–7, 145, 174, 180
  case histories 80–7
  image acquisition parameters 81
Cholinergic activity 145
Cingulate gyrus 138
Cognitive abilities 154
Cognitive functions 149
Cognitive problems 155
Cognitive tasks 164
Collimators 4–6, 34, 36, 41–3, 46, 47
Complex cognition 139
Computer-assisted X-ray tomography (CT scan) 7, 11, 13
Computer-generated neuropsychological maps 127
Contralateral parietal cortex 161
Control tasks 146
Corpus callosum 154
Correlation analysis 149, 155
Cortexplorer 150
Cortical areas activated by thinking 139
Cortical basal degeneration 71
Cortical lesions 138
Cortical myoclonus 177
Cosmological search 128
Criminal face 126
Cut-off frequency 32

Data analysis 149, 155, 174
Dementia 18, 58, 167
  need for proper diagnosis of aetiology of 58
  treatable and reversible causes of 58
Deoxyglucose 176
Depression 167, 178, 179
  case histories 87–91
  image acquisiton parameters 88, 89, 90
Dexamethasone suppression test (DST) 91
Directed attention 138, 139
Disease mechanisms 180
Distributed network 141
Dopamine 21
Dopamine-blocking agent 176
Dopamine function 176
Dopaminergic receptor systems 21
Dorsolateral posterior parietal cortex 138
Dorsolateral premotor prefrontal cortex 138
Dosage 47
Dual energy window 35
"dyadic hub and spoke" network 139

Electrical stimulation 127, 176, 177
Electroconvulsive therapy (ECT) 176
Electroencephalogram (EEG) 127
Electronic collimation 4
Emission tomography 5–7
  principles of 3

Energy resolution 35
Energy response 36
Epilepsy 124, 133, 176
  associated psychiatric aspects 113–15
  case histories 109–15
  image acquisition parameters 110, 111, 114
Epistemological search 128
Ethylene-cysteine-dimer (ECD) 19

Fahr's disease
  case history 104–5
  image acquisition parameters 105
FAS word generation protocol 165, 166
$^{18}$FDG 74, 134
Filtered back-projection 31
Filtering 32
  principles of 32
Finger-opposition task 160
Focal brain lesions 154
Focal hypoperfusion 175
Focal seizures 176
Fourier space 32
Fourier Transformation 32
Frequency space 32
Frontal activation task 162
Frontal blood flow 167
Frontal dementias 66, 179
Frontal eye fields 169
Frontal lobe 155, 168
Frontal lobe activation 162, 164, 165
Frontal lobe dementias 66–7, 179
  case history 66–7
  image acquisition parameters 66

GABA receptor system 21
$^{67}$Ga-citrate 14
Galenic theory 123
Gamma camera 4, 39
Gamma camera imaging 4
Gamma ray scattering 6
Gamma rays 3, 4, 35
Gantry system 37, 38
GE/CGR Neurocam 29, 157, 168
  acquisition protocols 43
  data sampling 43
  design and performance 40
  physical assessment 42
  planar sensitivity 42
  reconstructed resolution 43
  reconstruction protocol 44
  resolution 42
  sensitivity 42
  system planar resolution 43
  tomographic sensitivity 42
Geschwind syndrome 115
GE Star 3000 computer 41
Gilles de la Tourette syndrome (GTS)
  case histories 99–100
  image acquisition parameters 99

Glucose metabolic rate  144

Hallucinations  175, 176
Hexamethyl propylene amine oxime
    (HMPAO)  18, 19
HIPDM  16
Hippocampi  154
Human motor homunculus  159
Huntington's disease  178, 179
    case history  101–2
    image acquisition parameters  101
Hypertension  175
Hypoperfusion  175

$^{123}$I  26
$^{123}$I-flumazenil  13
$^{123}$I-HIPDM  13, 15
$^{123}$I-IBZM  13, 43, 176
$^{123}$I-IMP  13, 15, 146, 148, 154, 176
$^{123}$I-iodoantipyrine  15
$^{123}$I-IQNB  13
$^{123}$I-ketanserin  13
$^{123}$I-labelled amines  15
$^{123}$I-labelled human serum albumin (HSA)  14
Image quality  6
Imaging times  39
Inelastic scattering  35
Infantile autism  73–80
    case histories  73–80
    image acquisition parameters  74, 75
Inferior-temporal regions  154, 155
Intracerebral tumours  13
Intracranial haematomas  13
4-Iodoantipyrene  16
Ipsilateral cerebellar hemisphere activity  148
Ipsilateral medial frontal and parietal areas  155
Isotropic sampling  40
Iterative reconstruction  33

'k' factor  35

Language disorders  135
Learning process  137
Learning tasks  155
Left superior temporal/inferior parietal area  153
Lexical processing  141
Limited tomography  6
Local neural nets  139

Magnetic resonance imaging (MRI)  7, 11, 150
Malignancy
    case histories  106–9
    image acquisition parameters  106, 107, 108
Memory  154

Memory tasks  154
Mental activity  146
Metabolic activity  176
Middle frontal gyri  154
Mind–brain interaction  127
Monoamines  21
MOSE  15
Motor activation studies  145
Motor cortex  168
Motor tasks  158
Movement disorders  96, 161, 164
MRP20  19
Multi-detector single slice systems  148
Multi-detector systems  38, 46
Multi-detector/multi-head gamma camera  149
Multi-detector/multi-headed SPET  39, 46
Multi-focal neuronal systems  137
Multi-infarct dementia
    case histories  63–66
    image acquisition parameters  63, 64, 65
Multi-slice machines  6
Multiple images  173
Multiple processors  137
Multiple sclerosis
    case history  115–17
    image acquisition parameters  115
Muscarinic receptor system  21
Myocardial perfusion  5

NaI(Tl) crystal  4, 41
Narrow angle tomography  6
Nausea  175
Neural networks  136
Neuroactivation
    activation procedures  144
    choice of SPET instrument  148
    choice of tracer  147
    future applications  173, 178
    guide to performing studies  182
    methodological issues  144
    normal controls  153
    principles of  143
    procedures for  157
    protocol design  144
Neuroanatomy  51
Neurobiology  180
Neurocam. See GE/CGR Neurocam
Neurochemistry  180
Neuroimaging  51
Neurophysiological responses to
        pharmacological or behavioural stimuli  143
Neuropsychiatric diseases 173, 175, 179
Neuropsychiatric treatment evaluation  179
Neuropsychology  127
Neuroreceptor ligands  13, 25–6
Nickel poisoning  17
Nicotinic receptor system  21
Nitroglycerin  145

Normal neuroanatomy and neuroimaging  51
Normal pressure hydrocephalus  70–1
   image acquisition parameters  70
Nuclear magnetic resonance imaging (MRI scanning). *See* Magnetic resonance imaging

Obsessive–compulsive disorder
   case history  94–6
   image acquisition parameters  94
Occipital cortex  168, 170
Occipital lobe activation  168, 170
Occipital rCBF response  175
Occipital regions  155
Offpeak energy windows  35
Opioid receptor system  21
Osaka/Hitachi SPECT 2000  44
Oxygen-15  146

Panic attacks  167
Parallel distributed processing (PDP)  136–41
Parietal lobe activation  160
Parietal protocol  161
Parkinson's disease  178, 179
   case histories  96–8
   image acquisition parameters  97
Partial volume effect  34
Pediatric developmental disorders  73
Peptides  21
Perfusion tracers  13
PET  4, 6, 134, 143, 153, 173
   limitations of  149
   minimum detectable quantities  7
   radiation exposure  8
   radionuclides for  7
   radiopharmaceuticals for  7
   spatial resolution  8
pH shift gradient mechanism  15
Pharmacological activation studies  145
Photomultiplier tubes (PMTs)  4, 41
Photon deficiency  16
Photopeak windows  35
Phrenology  124
Picker PRISM  46
Pick's disease  179
Pineal gland  129
PIPSE  15
Planar emission imaging  4
Planning tasks  164
Plasma volume  14
Poisson statistics  6
Positron electron annihilation  3, 6
Positron emission tomography. *See* PET
Positron emitters  3
Pseudodementia  179
Psychiatric illnesses  87

Quality control  36

Radiation exposure  8
Radiation protection  8, 47
Radioactive tracers  11, 147
Radioisotopes, very short half-life  146
Radionuclide imaging  3
Radionuclides  3
   for PET  3
   for SPET  3
Radiopharmaceuticals  4, 6, 47
   BBB  13
   brain perfusion  14
   cerebral blood volume  14
   for PET  7
   for SPET  7
   receptors  21
Ramp  32
Ramp filter  32, 42
Receptors, radiopharmaceuticals  21
Reconstructed image quality  33
Reconstruction process  36, 37
Red blood cells (RBC)  14
Reductive materialism  130
Regional cerebral blood flow (rCBF)  51, 133, 139, 144, 150, 153, 174, 175
Regions of interest (ROI)  149, 153, 157
Right parahippocampal blood flow  167
Right temporal lobe  176

Sagittal images  166, 169, 171
Scatter compensation techniques  35
Scattering  35
Schizophrenia  144, 175, 179
   case histories  91–3
   image acquisition parameters  92
$^{75}$Se-labelled diamines  15
Senile dementia  18
Sensory tasks  168
Serial processing  138
Serotonin receptor system  21
Shimadzu Headtome SET-O31  44
Silent arithmetic calculation  146
Single detector systems  148
Single photon emission tomography (SPET). *See* SPET
Single photon emitters  3
Single rotating gamma camera  29
Single slice machines  6
SME810  45
Smoothing filter  32
Sodium diethyldithiocarbamate (NaDDC)  17
Sodium iodide NaI(Tl) scintillation crystal  4, 41
Sodium–potassium pump  14
Spatial resolution  34
Spatial response  36
Spatial sampling  34
SPECT. *See* SPET
SPET  4, 5, 143, 173
   choice of instrument  148
   instrumentation  29

limitations of 149
minimum detectable quantities 9
quality control 36
radiation exposure 8
radionuclides for 3
radiopharmaceuticals for 7
resolution 173
spatial resolution 8
Stannous chloride 14
Statistical approach 149
Striate cortex 153
Stroboscopic stimulation 153
Stroke 16, 80, 126, 161, 164, 175, 180
Stroop protocol 26, 164
Superior frontal gyri 154
Sydenham's chorea
case history 102–4
image acquisition parameters 102
Synaptic connections 138
Synaptic junction 137

Tactile hallucinations 175
Talairach stereotactic atlas 150
Task performance, effects of pathological states on 139
$^{99m}$Tc 4, 14, 26, 146
$^{99m}$Tc-BATO-2MP 13
$^{99m}$Tc-brain agents 20
$^{99m}$Tc-DTPA 12, 13
$^{99m}$Tc-ECD 13, 21
$^{99m}$Tc-GH 12, 13
$^{99m}$Tc-HMPAO 13, 18, 19, 28–31, 33, 35, 38, 41, 43, 45, 47, 51, 52, 54, 56, 58, 59, 60, 63, 64, 68, 147, 148, 153–5, 157, 161, 168, 174, 175, 176, 177
$^{99m}$Tc-L,L-ECD 18
$^{99m}$Tc-labelled cerebral perfusion agents 20
$^{99m}$Tc-labelled human serum albumin (HSA) 14
$^{99m}$Tc-labelled tracers 17
$^{99m}$Tc-MRP20 18

$^{99m}$Tc-pertechnetate 12
Temporal lobe epilepsy 177
Thallium intoxication 17
Thinking
cortical areas activated by 139
processes involved in 139
Thinking tasks 146, 164
$^{201}$Tl-chloride 5, 12, 14, 17
$^{201}$Tl-DDC 17
Tomographic data acquisition 29
Toshiba GCA-9300A 46
Transaxial images 167, 170
Transient ischaemic attacks (TIAs) 4, 145, 175
Trephining 123
Trionix TRIAD 46
Tumours 126, 138

Vascular reactivity 175
Vertebrobasilar insufficiency 145, 175
Vertigo 175
Vision processes 168
Visual activation task 168
Visual cortex 153, 154
Visual imagery 154
Visual pathway 168
Visuomotor learning 155
Volumetric dynamic SPET 40
Volumetric imaging 40
Voluntary eye movements 170, 171

Wilson's disease 17
Wisconsin Card Sort test 144

Xenon-133 134, 139, 144, 146–9
X-ray computed tomography (CT scan). *See* Computer-assisted X-ray tomography (CT scan)